Empowered Healing

Creating Quality of Life While Journeying with Cancer

Susanne M. Alexander and Craig A. Farnsworth

Foreword by Dr. Annaliisa McGlinn

Testimonials

There is a pattern to the personality of long-term survivors. They demonstrate action, wisdom, and devotion in their response to cancer and seek personal empowerment. *Empowered Healing* coaches and helps you to create a quality of life that gives your body the message to live. When you love your life, your body shows its love too.

~ Bernie Siegel, MD, best-selling author of *Love, Medicine & Miracles*, *Faith, Hope & Healing* and *Help Me to Heal*, **www.berniesiegelmd.com**

Empowered Healing is a remarkable resource for people who are dealing with a loved one/friend who has been diagnosed with the disease of cancer, especially a cancer that is long term. I am impressed with the insights and tools provided for those on such a journey.

~ Thenice Gall, American Cancer Society board of directors, Akron, Ohio, Chapter

I am very touched by this work and your thoroughness. I feel this book will help many and not just those with cancer. Great work.

~ Karen Schulman, photographic artist, owner of Focus Adventures, and breast cancer survivor

This is a helpful tool, with much practical information, helpful encouragement, and lovely personal stories.

~ Eileen Coan, MA, MLS, medical librarian, The Gathering Place, **www.touchedbycancer.org**

Empowered Healing is a superb read, heartfelt, and practical. It is a testimonial on becoming an authentic human being, which is one who assesses their circumstances or situation, makes a decision, and takes responsibility for it. I feel emboldened to continue the path I have chosen to pursue as I continue to live with the results of a lymphoma. I can affirm that many practical suggestions you offer work—at least for me in my circumstance. Others I had not tried but will incorporate within my routine. The range of your approach in your book offers both the pragmatist and the idealist a considerable range of options to incorporate in their life's healing journey. While the locus of *Empowered Healing* grew from the authors' co-journey with cancer, this book provides guidance, suggestions, and practices that can be applied to a variety of life-challenging experiences anyone may face on a daily basis. *Empowered Healing* shines a loving beacon of light and truth in mind and heart and allows us to walk the healing path with conscious dignity, honesty, care, gratitude, and enthusiasm.

~ Reggie Newkirk, author, diversity/equity trainer, motivational speaker, youth development coach, and lymphoma patient

Empowered Healing

Version: August 2012
Published in English by Marriage Transformation LLC
Chattanooga, Tennessee, USA
www.marriagetransformation.com;;
Susanne@marriagetransformation.com

International Standard Book Number/ISBN: 978-0-9816666-6-2

© 2012 Marriage Transformation LLC. All international rights reserved for the book as a whole. No part of this book may be reproduced by any mechanical, photographic, or electronic process, or by any other means, in the form of a photographic or digital recording, nor may it be stored in a retrieval system, transmitted, or otherwise copied for public or private use, including on the Internet, or resold, without the written permission of Marriage Transformation, except by a reviewer, who may quote brief passages in a review. Translations into other languages also require permission. *Thank you for respecting this legal copyright. Your integrity with this process spreads a spirit of loving respect throughout the world and makes us very happy.*

This publication is intended to provide helpful and educational information about responding to cancer. It is sold with the understanding that the publisher and the authors are not engaged in rendering legal, clinical, or medical advice. No information, advice, or suggestions by the authors are intended to take the place of directly consulting with a medical or therapy professional. If expert assistance is required, the services of a competent licensed professional should be sought. The authors and publisher shall have neither liability nor responsibility to any person or entity with respect to any loss or damage caused, or alleged to be caused, directly or indirectly, by the information contained in this book.

Cover Design: Jeff Duckworth (**www.duckofalltrades.com**)

Dedication

To Lu and Bob Farnsworth:
Thank you for the gift of your son Craig
to my life, his family, and the world.
With love,
Susanne

Appreciation

Many people have helped with reviewing and giving feedback on *Empowered Healing* and contributed their expertise, support, and encouragement. Much appreciation to Roger Bascom, Shirley Bascom, Barry Bittman, Karen Bittman, Debbie Boyd Tressler, Dan Clark, Eileen Coan, Jennifer DeMaria, Thenice Gall, Arlene Nedd Green, Linda Gruenspan, Ellen Heyman, Bronwyn Jones, Kimberly Klein, Janet Lyon, Brenda Maxwell Zografov MD, AnnaLiisa McGlinn MD, Ed Muttart, Reggie Newkirk, Karen Schulman, Bernie Siegel MD, Michelle Farnsworth Tashakor, Holly Timberlake, Nancy Tolles, and Nik Tressler.

The staff and the volunteers at the Gathering Place (**www.touchedbycancer.org**) provided us amazing ongoing support, and their workshop on brain tumors provided the impetus for the creation of this book. The staff of University Hospitals of Cleveland (**www.uhhospitals.org**) were wonderful in partnering with us for Craig's treatment and care. The staff of Hospice of the Western Reserve (**www.hospicewr.org**) was the absolute best team we could have had. Much appreciation to you all.

What is the Purpose of *Empowered Healing*?

This is a practical guide to empowered personal responsibility in healing and creating quality of life while experiencing cancer. It is primarily designed to help patients, especially those who are married. It also provides caregivers with new and effective tools for patient support and for their own well-being. Caregivers is a broad term that includes family members or hired personnel. The book may also be helpful for those concerned about a cancer patient, even if they are not involved in direct patient care, such as medical personnel and friends.

Globally, according to the World Health Organization, cancer kills millions of people each year. And the American Cancer Society says Americans face a 30–50 percent chance of developing cancer in their lifetime. Even for those who do not develop cancer, they still interact with family members or friends who are struggling to respond to this diagnosis. This is a disease that touches most people's lives.

Most cancer patients search for an often-elusive cure or miracle treatment. Some choose to simply let the disease progress. Many choose multiple treatment options that are challenging in their side effects. However, whatever the type of cancer and whatever treatment choices a patient and family make, maintaining empowered personal responsibility in responding to the diagnosis, healing, and in creating optimum quality of life is vital.

Making excellent choices and establishing goals for maintaining quality of life is a team exploration with a patient, caregiver/family, and medical staff. *Empowered Healing* guides patients and their loved ones through a systematic fact-based, spirit-guided approach. The choices involved in this approach can potentially lengthen cancer patient's lives and also help them increase the quality of the time they have, no matter how long it is.

This approach to cancer grew out of the authors' own experiences with Craig Farnsworth's cancer diagnosis and his wife's caregiving (Susanne M. Alexander). Susanne is an experienced writer and journalist. Craig knew from the moment of his tumor diagnosis that his approach was going to be different from the way most people would respond. He was then further inspired by Dr. Bernie Siegel's description of being an exceptional cancer patient in his book *Love, Medicine, and Miracles*. Susanne also did her best to be an exceptional caregiver. As a result, Craig lived far longer than expected with excellent quality of life throughout. This book unfolded weeks before Craig's passing under hospice care.

www.marriagetransformation.com/store_EmpoweredHealing.htm

Contents

FOREWORD 1
THE CONTEXT 4
THE GOAL 9
PART 1: THE FACT-BASED CHOICES 13
   1 - Focus on Being Realistic 14
   2 - Seek Knowledge 17
   3 - Speak Up 22
   4 - Maximize Certainty 25
   5 - Choose Integrated Treatment 28
   6 - Create a Team 31
   7 - Improve the Process 35
   8 - Ask for Help 39
   9 - Choose Where to Be 43
   10 - Communicate Well 46

PART 2: THE SPIRIT-GUIDED CHOICES 51
   1 - Engage in Prayer 52
   2 - Meditate and Visualize 55
   3 - Seek Inspiration 59
   4 - Experience the Arts 62
   5 - Strive to Be Your Best 66
   6 - Serve Others 69
   7 - Build Unity 72
   8 - Expand Love 76
   9 - Feel Happy 80
   10 - Die (and Live) Consciously 84

RE-VISITING EMPOWERMENT 89
APPENDICES
   A: Copy of "Three Tools of Healing" Poster 91
   B: Empowering Character Qualities 92
ABOUT THE AUTHORS 99
PLEASE CONTACT US 101

Foreword – Annaliisa McGlinn, MD, Radiation Oncologist

As a Radiation Oncologist, most people think that what I do is treat people with high energy x-rays in an attempt to provide a cure or to provide symptom relief for improving quality of life. But what I really do is listen, teach, and try to guide patients into living beyond their cancer. What I love about my job is the human interaction, the opportunity to provide comfort and inspire people.

When my patients meet me, I have two goals: 1) By the end of the clinic visit, they understand their diagnosis and the rationale for the treatment options, including benefits and potential side effects; 2) I've opened the door for the patient and families to live beyond the cancer.

After we finish discussing the diagnosis and treatment, I will ask about how they are coping mentally, as well as how their interpersonal relationships have been affected with spouses, kids, and friends. I let patients know that the range of emotions they are experiencing is normal. By talking about their cancer, their body energy is freed up for healing, and their immune system is elevated to fight the cancer, rather than them spending the body's energy stuffing the emotions inside. I encourage patients to address the elephant in the room and have the tough conversations with their loved ones, tears and all, because this will bring them closer together and provide a sense of relief. Why is this? Because then each person affected by the diagnosis—patient and loved ones—feel a bond and connection rather than isolation while trying to protect the other. Knowing how hard it is to have these conversations across the kitchen table, I often recommend that patients and loved ones take short walks—as long as the patient is physically able.

I recommend patients examine stressful relationships and try to heal them, even if it means agreeing to disagree and go separate ways in peace. Again, this frees up energy for healing, and elevates the immune system.

I recommend patients do something every day that promotes a sense of well-being, which ultimately promotes a sense of inner peace and rest. This is defined differently for each patient. Is it music? Reaching out and speaking with an old friend? Watching birds? Looking at the garden? Playing with the grandkids or kids? This is self-affirming and again stimulates the immune system to help fight the cancer.

I believe in the power of prayer. For those patients that believe in a Higher Power, however defined, I encourage them to pray.

With each new patient, I talk about all of this and more, whether or not our intent is for cure or to treat symptoms to promote quality of life.

During my time as a Radiation Oncologist, I have met many patients who have done better than one would expect. Uniformly, they all made changes in their lives that promoted love, communication, self-affirmation, and affirmation of others. These patients universally were able to use humor, allowed the tears to flow, and did the mental processing required with the diagnosis of cancer.

I'm grateful for what my patients have taught me and the practices that I've learned from Dr. Bernie Siegel (*Love, Medicine, and Miracles*) that I use every day. *Empowered Healing* is in the spirit of his work, and it will guide patients through claiming their emotions, being empowered in responding to their diagnoses, and helping them and their families strive for quality of life.

AnnaLiisa McGlinn, MD

Dr. McGlinn is the Director of Radiation Oncology at the Yolanda G. Barco Oncology Institute in Meadville Medical Center, Meadville, Pennsylvania. This facility is an integrative cancer treatment center that was founded on the holistic principles that Bernie Siegel, MD, and Barry Bittman, MD, have pioneered for many years.

— *Foreword* —

Note: If you are aware of a cancer-related organization that may wish to use this book as a fundraising tool, please connect them to Marriage Transformation.

The websites are:

www.marriagetransformation.com/store_EmpoweredHealing.htm,
www.marriagetransformation.com.

You can also reach Susanne at
Susanne@marriagetransformation.com.

Craig's blog: **www.factbasedspiritguidedpath.blogspot.com**

The Context:
A FRAMEWORK FOR EMPOWERED HEALING

Once you begin traveling with cancer, whether you are the person with the diagnosis or you are a loved one, the term "quality of life" becomes a part of your everyday world. You may be striving to maintain the quality you had before the diagnosis and treatments began, or you may be creating new definitions of what quality looks like at each stage of the journey. This book lays out the tools we developed and used on our own journey with cancer. As you fully use them, you can be inspired to have a high-quality life, as we had.

Responding to Cancer

In the summer of 2007, Craig had a tumor removed from the left parietal lobe of his brain, the area that controls motor skills. It was subsequently diagnosed as Glioblastoma Multiforme, a highly aggressive form of primary cancer. From the first hour of the news that he had a tumor in his brain, he focused on the facts of his circumstance and refused to "descend into speculation, worry, and anxiety." Over the subsequent weeks, he began to formulate how he wanted to respond to his diagnosis and entitled it the "fact-based, spirit-guided approach." He then invited his wife, Susanne, to join with him in her role as caregiver.

It was not until the last period of Craig's life, in the spring of 2009, that we began to systematically write down our understanding of the components of this approach. We reflected on and reviewed what we had successfully done during Craig's cancer journey, and we recorded what we learned in the process. We hope that our experience now benefits you. Throughout this book, you will hear Craig's voice as one responding to a cancer diagnosis and Susanne's voice as the caregiver. However, we have made efforts to keep our suggestions broad enough to apply across a wide range of cancers, not simply brain cancer as Craig experienced.

Our attitude was that life is a continuous process of personal growth and transformation. Cancer is like any test or difficulty in life—it can be an opportunity to engage in this process. A vital component of the fact-based, spirit-guided approach is that scientific, spiritual, and emotional factors must work in harmony. It is then possible to achieve maximum personal growth, healing, and quality of life. We regard healing as a process that is only partially physical. Much of Craig's healing involved relationships, his soul, and his emotions. We believe our approach extended Craig's physical life and definitely improved its quality. We also saw ourselves as empowered advocates for Craig's well-being, and both of us were fully involved as marriage partners in making whatever choices arose.

Overview of the Integrated Fact-Based, Spirit-Guided Approach

When faced with symptoms or a diagnosis for any medical condition, our automatic responses of denial, anger, or anxiety tend to kick in. A diagnosis of cancer, in particular, seems to fill us with dread. The fact-based aspects of this integrated approach help you focus on the known information available to you, rather than descending into a mire of emotions that shut off your rational brain. Part 1 includes guidance about holding tight to the facts about a given aspect of life, instead of imaginary worries, to achieve a level of serenity.

When the facts are particularly difficult or unclear, then the spirit-guided choices in Part 2 provided here are available to help you respond effectively. The guidance includes mental, emotional, and spiritual aspects. This part of the approach to empowered healing includes the belief that there is a natural impulse inside each person to reach for the good, to pray or converse with God or a Higher Power in some fashion, and to seek answers from spiritual sources. In part, we communicate the view that you are a spiritual being having physical experiences. The approach involves reaching for new answers, choosing new words to say and actions to take, and seeking further guidance than is available from the facts. The intent from using this approach is to empower you to live as fully as possible.

For the purpose of clarity and learning, we have laid out the choices of the "fact-based approach" and the "spirit-guided approach" separately. However, they are anything but separate. This is actually an *integrated process*, where both approaches happen together, and the tools of each intermingle. You may not choose to use all of the ideas presented if they are not a fit for you. However, you will likely discover that the more of them you use, the more empowered you will feel.

Why Include Character Qualities?

A unique feature of this book is the inclusion of character qualities that you may find helpful to practice for successful use of this approach. Both of us were trained as relationship and marriage coaches with a specialty in character development, so we include some of our work on this subject. We firmly believe that it enhances healing and well-being when people speak and act in positive ways, regardless of what challenges they are facing. (See Appendix B for more detail.)

Why "Empowered Healing"?

When faced with a major difficulty, we can be tempted at times to ignore it or let others make decisions for us. We can be especially tempted to automatically delegate responsibility and leadership for our healing to doctors, rather than staying in charge of our own selves and working in partnership with our medical team and loved ones. This book is about empowering you to be in charge of, as much as possible, your healing process. As Dr. Bernie Siegel says in his books *Peace, Love & Healing* and *Help Me to Heal* (coauthored with Yosaif August), *you are a "respant," a responsible participant.*

An illness may be a sign that you are out of balance in your body or life in some way, and you now have the opportunity to examine your whole life for where you need healing. This book is about being powerful with your choices and maximizing your ability to heal holistically from cancer. It is not about creating remission or a cure, although that may be the outcome of your choices. It is an invitation to systematically take steps that make the maximum amount of healing and quality of life possible to occur.

What Are You Committed to Creating in Your Life?

Taking the fact-based, spirit-guided approach to cancer involves making a commitment to empowered healing. It is making a commitment to create maximum quality of life—however you define that. Practicing "commitment" involves making and keeping a reasonable promise or binding agreement to oneself or to others. If making powerful commitments is not how you have previously approached problems in your life, it may be a significant shift to try a new way.

Whether this is a new approach for you or more familiar, be patient, gentle, and kind with yourself and your loved ones as you assess and choose how you want to heal. Know that you will do well with what you choose at times, and at other times trip or fall. Sometimes it will be two steps forward and only one back. Other times you will feel as if you are standing still and not making progress. You may race ahead instead and do very well. You may question whether you can commit to healing and well-being—it may seem like too much work—but it is worth it. These qualities will help:

Patience is maintaining steady awareness and control of one's thoughts and responses while waiting for or seeking an outcome; controlling one's words and actions while willingly and calmly taking the time to respond to difficult, inconvenient, hurtful, delaying, or troublesome situations.

Gentleness is expressing consideration from the heart, honoring the feelings of others and oneself, and using soft and careful physical touch, movement, and words.

Kindness is considering the needs or wants of others and acting in a deliberately warm-hearted and empathetic manner to meet them.

Dr. Bernie Siegel also writes in his book *Love, Medicine, and Miracles* about the choice of being an exceptional cancer patient. For us, the tools we share with you in *Empowered Healing* helped us create an exceptional cancer journey. What are you committed to creating in your life?

The choice is yours:

You can choose everything, even acceptance
   Choosing takes courage
      Choosing eliminates blaming
         Choosing creates power
            Choosing creates new outcomes
               Choosing creates miracles

With love,
Susanne M. Alexander and Craig A. Farnsworth

The Goal of the Fact-Based, Spirit-Guided Approach:
LIVE A HIGH-QUALITY LIFE

The Concept

Throughout your experience with cancer, we encourage you to continually evaluate the quality of your life. Before you engage in treatment options, consider how they may affect your *whole* life, not only whether the treatment *extends* your life. Cancer and its treatments tend to affect your body, mind, and emotions. Achieving quality includes assessing your ability to work, play with your children or grandchildren, drive, exercise, spend time with friends, participate in spiritual activities, and more. Striving for a high-quality life will require flexibility on your part—sometimes it will be possible to achieve, and sometimes you won't quite make it. However, it is worth the effort…one day at a time.

It is wise to consciously identify and communicate what counts as "quality" for you overall and at specific times. Your view of it may change as your circumstances and your body's response to the disease and treatments change. Your definition of "quality" may also be very different from that of your family, friends, medical staff, or spiritual leaders, so it is important that they know *your* definition. Sometimes others may have to make decisions on your behalf that affect the quality of your life, and your input is vital to guide them.

Quality usually includes living your life as fully as possible while maintaining balance and health for you and your support team. However, it can also include doing specific actions or simply doing whatever you would normally do if cancer or treatments were not present. Consider that the *quality* of your life is potentially just as important, if not more so, than the *quantity* of time you have left to live. One of the interesting outcomes of creating quality is that it may also extend your life. You become more focused on living happily than on prognosis statistics that are unlikely to be an exact match for you.

To maximize your quality of life, consider *integrating* both the fact-based and spirit-guided aspects in responding to cancer and healing. Using them together will increase your empowerment with making effective choices.

Personal Perspectives

Craig: My oncologist and I agreed throughout my treatment and recovery that quality of life was vital. As I considered all the worst possible outcomes, I came to the conclusion that my passing away would not be the worst. For me, it would be most difficult living for months or even years in a severely impaired state with a terrible quality of life. However, I noticed that how I defined "quality" changed as my condition changed. Even when I was impaired physically and mentally, if I could maintain contact with family and friends and find enjoyable or useful activities, I was okay. What I noticed, as well, was that no matter what happened physically, I could still pray, and that was a key quality indicator for me.

It was a continual adventure trying to maintain the quality of my physical life. I evaluated treatment options, choosing some. At times, I declined ones that would interfere too much with life. Surgeries often seemed to occur as emergencies, and I wish I had done a better job of having discussions with the surgeon ahead of time about their possible impact on the quality of my functioning. Managing medications and supplements was another area of constant adjustment and at times experimentation, as I worked with my doctors and caregivers to maximize health and reduce symptoms from the treatments and spread of the tumor.

I enhanced the quality of my mental and emotional life with the support of family, friends, and many other resources. I requested that sick friends not visit, but I didn't isolate myself, as I believed enjoying the visitors enhanced my immune system strength. I was confident that the happiness I felt from having visitors was very healing. As I began in-home hospice care, I included music and art therapy to enhance the quality of my time and help me process the emotions of that stage. At that point, quality for me became days when there was more to be grateful for than to complain about!

The quality of my spiritual life expanded and grew throughout the whole journey, as I increased the amount of prayer, meditation, and visualization I did. I continually adjusted my participation in spiritual activities, but stayed involved throughout.

Susanne: My goal throughout my husband's cancer journey was to identify and facilitate whatever enhanced his quality of life. This meant such actions as: encouraging and coordinating visits, messages, and phone calls from family and friends; supporting him working and staying in touch with coworkers; taking him places outside of our home; adjusting our home environment for comfort, safety, and to support well-being; picking up library materials; cooking nutritious and favorite foods; and learning to do my husband's usual tasks well enough that he would no longer worry about them getting done.

It became clear to me along the way that it was important to my husband's happiness that I also take care of myself and maintain quality of life for me as well. The medical establishment focuses on the patient and not much on the well-being of the caretaker, so it was up to me to make good choices. Caring friends and relatives regularly reminded me that I could best help my husband if I took care of myself. This empowered me to take naps, rest, exercise, and eat well.

I attended my own support group, listened to relaxation recordings, prayed, received regular massages, and took respite days while a friend stayed in our home. I facilitated spiritual groups in our home, and I also made time to enjoy occasional meals out with close friends. I requested family and friends to keep our home supplied with beautiful flowers to uplift my spirits, and they did so. I did grieving work with the help of others as each loss or change occurred. Through all these efforts, I stayed in much better shape physically, mentally, emotionally, and spiritually than I ever dreamed was possible.

Practice in Action

Ask yourself regularly whether you are making choices that enhance your quality of life, and step into action to change direction as needed.

Beneficial Character Strengths

Enthusiasm is expressing genuine positive and joyful feelings, often in a high-spirited way, about an occasion, activity, important occurrence, goal, person, or extraordinary situation.

Flexibility is adjusting to life as it happens and embracing changes as needed, while remaining true to one's core values, beliefs, and appropriate priorities.

Part 1: The Fact-Based Choices

Note: The Fact-Based Choices here in Part 1 are ideally *integrated* in action with Part 2, the Spirit-Guided Choices.

1 - Fact-Based Choice:
FOCUS ON BEING REALISTIC

The Concept

Whether you are at the beginning of your cancer journey or farther along, you probably have a mix of emotions and events happening. Denial and resistance are common responses to a diagnosis of cancer or when tests results come back with difficult news. Some of this response is a normal and natural way that you protect yourself from what is very painful to face. It gives you time to grieve and adjust to reality. However, when you carry denial to excess, or bury yourself in it for too long, conditions can worsen, treatment options can be lost, and opportunities for help from others can be postponed or missed.

Being realistic requires self-discipline and deep honesty with yourself. When you understand and accept the reality of your current circumstances and conditions, without either exaggerating how bad they are or denying the challenges, it helps you avoid speculation, anxiety, and worry. True acceptance of your situation actually creates a greater opportunity for you to feel hope for a good outcome. It also puts you in charge of taking the actions needed for the well-being of your body, heart, mind, and soul. It becomes possible for you to be the leader of determining your treatment plan.

It can be helpful to watch the words you use in describing what is occurring. You can say you have received a "diagnosis of cancer," or that you are "experiencing cancer at this time," rather than saying you "*have* cancer". When you say you "have cancer," it can seem like permanent ownership and that the disease is a permanent resident in your body. The words you use can indicate you are not denying what is happening, and you are open to what the future may be.

Personal Perspectives

Craig: When I received the diagnosis that I had a tumor, before I even knew that it was cancerous, I had a calm inner sense that I should maintain my focus on the facts of what I knew. I was grateful for the honesty of my doctors. At that point, the verifiable facts included a golf-ball sized tumor that was swelling in a location in my brain that was consistent with all the right-side motor symptoms I was experiencing. This focus helped me to not get into speculating or worrying. From that place, I was able to consider joy and laughter as a possibility in coping with what was to come. I requested extensive help with this approach from my family and friends, asking for prayers, visits, and phone calls.

Denial wasn't initially an issue for me. However, after the tumor was removed, I believed for a long time that cancer was gone and no longer a problem. I almost felt as if I was humoring the doctors by going along with radiation and chemotherapy. It took a few months and further test results for me to be more realistic and accept that I was still dealing with active cancer growth.

As I met with my doctors, I began to realize that I needed to be in charge of what happened to my body. The choices for surgery, chemotherapy, and radiation, as well as for whether I did or did not use unconventional treatments were mine. I chose to make decisions in consultation with others, but I was the leader.

Susanne: Focusing on the facts does help me minimize anxiety, but I also recognized that understanding my feelings was a legitimate part of searching for the facts. I found it helpful to examine and accept the worst that could happen and then work backwards to a more open and hopeful frame of mind. I was then calmer and more able to take effective action as well. For me this was not speculating about the future but empowering me to act powerfully in the present to create the best future outcomes.

Practice in Action

When circumstances change, ask yourself, "What are the facts?" Then identify what information is missing and a strategy for obtaining it and responding to the situation effectively.

Beneficial Character Strengths

Acceptance is a deep, meaningful embracing of who someone is, as well as acknowledging that people and events are as they are, or were as they were, rather than wasting time and energy trying to change people, regret the past, or influence events when it is unwise or there is no possibility of success.

Self-Discipline is maintaining the inner control to perform needed and important tasks; fulfill one's commitments, goals, and life purposes; and resist what is harmful to others or oneself.

2 - Fact-Based Choice: *SEEK KNOWLEDGE*

The Concept

With the cancer diagnosis, you are facing a new situation. Even if a relative or friend of yours has had cancer, or even if you have had cancer previously, this is now a new opportunity to expand your knowledge. The desire to search for knowledge begins with caring about yourself and wanting to do whatever you can that is needed to affect the course of the disease and your future.

To begin, determine what is vital information for decision-making that aids and empowers you. Assess what sources you trust and which you will ignore. As information comes to you, it will be important to discern what is useless or what to set aside for another time or stage in the process. It is also wise to determine what amount of information and on what topic is important for you. For instance, some people prefer to know less about the disease and more about the treatments.

While you will search for general knowledge about the disease, it is also wise to focus on what is case-specific for you. This could include obtaining your diagnosis, test results, and instructions for follow-up care in writing. Be aware, however, that you may not be able to effectively understand the medical terminology in any reports you obtain. You will likely have to seek assistance from others with training in reading and interpreting the results.

— *Empowered Healing* —

Your doctors will likely be willing to help you sort out and understand what information you are finding, and your primary oncologist is a key partner in this process. Medical librarians can also be of significant assistance. Your loved ones may be able to help you as well.

Here are some guidelines that may help your information search:

1. Seek wisely for answers and utilize as broad a range of resources and resource people as makes sense for you and your circumstances.
2. Read books and study current research on both conventional and unconventional medicine and healing methods. Obtain assistance where possible from specialists and medical librarians in choosing what to read and in understanding the content. Remember that information in books may already be several years old.
3. Determine whether you regard as useful the anecdotal stories from others about what worked for them. Try to talk directly with the person who had the experience.
4. Use the Internet in the process of searching for information, but ask librarians and your doctor(s) for reliable, accurate, and research-based websites, and verify all information obtained.
5. Ask questions and make notes on the answers to fully understand the disease, what is happening, and why.
6. Find out your family history of cancer and ask for help from genetic specialists to determine whether your diagnosis and family history may affect other family members.
7. Understand the clinical trials (experimental treatments) available to you and the implications for your safety and well-being of participating. Trials are often available at different research phases. Generally, Phase 1 is

— *Seek Knowledge* —

the first human group to go through safety and side-effect testing; Phase 2 is effectiveness testing; Phase 3 is testing and monitoring with a larger test group and comparing it to commonly used treatment; and Phase 4 is further information gathering. Consider carefully any randomized test where you may receive a placebo rather than an actual treatment.

8. Seek explanations of medical terminology.
9. Obtain all appropriate medical test results and other reports on a timely basis.
10. Analyze and understand test results with the help of highly skilled and educated experts.
11. Understand the limitations of medical equipment, treatments, and tests.

Personal Perspectives

Craig: We found a cancer support center near us that had a medical librarian and extensive resources. It was helpful to learn more about my body and begin to understand the terminology the doctors were using as they discussed my test results. We were frustrated in the beginning trying to even get the proper spelling for my diagnosis. Getting it in writing would have helped. Whenever we had a concern about a test, we obtained the report in writing so we could study it and then ask further questions.

We learned over time that while testing equipment and technology are often helpful, re results were still not able to tell us everything we really wanted to know. We also learned that we often had to practice patience while waiting for information. Sometimes we could obtain test results directly from the doctor; at other times, we had to request them through a medical records department. At times, the doctor had results immediately, and at other times, the doctor had to wait along with us. Whenever the wait seemed as if it was becoming too long, however, we called to ensure the report wasn't lost or sitting unread, or that our request for information was not misplaced.

Susanne: When the diagnosis first came, the amount of information that we needed to obtain and understand quickly was overwhelming. We relied on friends who were cancer patients to help us find what was most helpful and accurate. We purchased a 600-page report about my husband's specific cancer and treatment options to minimize the amount of research we had to do. It was helpful information, but it also filled my head with a lot of choices and scary statistics. Knowing the odds against my husband living more than a few months felt like an overwhelming burden. It was a challenge to feel optimistic. However, I was also encouraged by the various treatments that could make a difference for him. Our inquiry focused on what could extend his life with the least negative effect on the quality of his life. It was not an easy puzzle to solve.

As time went on, we had to go back into knowledge-seeking mode to learn about clinical trial options, the experience of recurrence, and hospice care. At times, my husband could do his own research, but often he needed me to help. Completing document request forms was always my job!

We learned that we could use the time while waiting for reports for purposes that were more productive than worrying about what they might say. We created plans and outlined choices that fit good or poor test outcomes. We strengthened our marriage relationship with activities and communication. We caught up with work or with what needed to be done around our home. There remained a low-level of anxiety, but it was more manageable when we kept busy.

— *Seek Knowledge* —

Practice in Action

Ask someone to evaluate the information you have gathered and help you to determine whether you understand what you have found or whether you need additional assistance.

Beneficial Character Strengths

Caring is giving sincere love, attention, consideration, and assistance to others and responding to needy situations in timely and appropriate ways.

Purposefulness is pursuing meaningful goals and participating in vital activities with determination.

3 - Fact-Based Choice:
SPEAK UP

The Concept

Speaking up to obtain the facts related to your diagnosis and treatment options puts you in the seat of personal power. Medical personnel will then know you are serious about wanting to be active with your situation. This concept includes advocating on your behalf for the best care, when test results are too slow, and when you need more information than is automatically provided to you. The more you feel that you have a voice in what is happening to you, then the greater will be your feeling of empowerment. You will have some control in a situation that at times can feel very out of your control.

Busy medical personnel can find it difficult to remember you and those who accompany you through your medical adventures. It is helpful for you to collect business cards and call people by name and ensure that those working with you use your name as well. You and/or your caregiver will have to track your requests for information and your needs and ensure that they are met. This is particularly important when you are in situations such as emergency rooms, where constantly changing priorities can cause delays and tasks to be missed inadvertently. Carrying a notebook at all times during medical visits can be very helpful. You can note both your questions and the answers.

Personal Perspectives

Craig: From the beginning, I insisted that the doctors fully disclose what was happening and what my options were. I wanted to know the facts. I was an active participant in making decisions with the doctors about the timing of tests. It was helpful to see actual images of what was occurring, so at times we went through the extra effort to move me to where I could see a computer screen and view MRI brain scan results.

I had regrets along the journey when I didn't ask for a second opinion or inquire about the possible outcomes for my choices. I rarely asked about prognosis or statistics, because that just seemed to be a guessing game that looked at the numerical averages for average people. I decided I had no wish to have anyone considering me as "average"!

Susanne: I was often my husband's second voice and the one who chased after test results. I tracked his medications and monitored his side effects. In emergency rooms, I made sure he could have food or ate as needed and that he got pain medication when appropriate. I also made sure I took breaks and got food for myself. Once he was admitted, I monitored his tests and medications, talking to the doctors, nurses, and other personnel as needed to ensure he received the care he needed.

I made requests for information from the doctors whenever it seemed helpful, including asking for blood test results to be faxed to us as soon as they were available. Yes, we then had to learn to interpret them, but I found that they informed me about what foods could help my husband improve his results (after I spoke up and got help from the staff nutritionist!).

Practice in Action

Stay calm and courteous, but make direct requests as needed. Be insistent even when told your request is unreasonable, if it is very important to you.

Beneficial Character Strengths

Assertiveness is speaking up or acting decisively to improve a situation for the benefit of others and oneself.

Confidence is trusting one's inner value, worthy intentions, capacity to think and act effectively, and ability to accomplish stated goals of oneself and of others.

4 - Fact-Based Choice: *MAXIMIZE CERTAINTY*

The Concept

The goal when making decisions is to ensure that you make the best ones for you. You want to maximize or establish certainty about the likely effectiveness of your choices as much as you can. This requires knowing as many of the facts as possible before deciding. You and your doctors together will decide how much information is useful to you and when it is helpful or not to have your medical team members speculate about a test result or symptoms.

A fact generally is something that can be proven as being accurate. However, it can also include the feelings you are experiencing. It can be a fact that you are angry or happy about something.

Assess how quickly you actually need to make decisions and avoid making them out of desperation. Sleep on your choices whenever possible, and re-visit them the next day or for as long as needed to maximize certainty. Keep in mind that specialists will have varied viewpoints and preferences, such as a surgeon to do surgery or a radio-oncologist to administer radiation. Remember that there are no absolute right answers with cancer and its treatment options. You can only make the wisest choices based on the best information available in the moment. When certainty is not possible, then the Spirit-Guided Choices in Part 2 may assist you.

Personal Perspectives

Craig: I studied Physics in college, and my work in the previous 30 years was in research and development, product management, and technical sales, so I was pretty darned good at sorting out the essential information. The engineer in me obviously wanted to measure, touch, and feel the truth. However, I also struggled at times with anxiety and frustration when the facts were unclear due to limitations in medical equipment and testing options, or we received misinformation.

At each phase of the cancer journey, I simply tried to find out as much as possible, consult with my wife and others, and then we made the best decisions we could.

Susanne: We often felt certain about our decisions about treatments but uncertain about what was really happening inside my husband's body. I often wished that the tools I have seen in science fiction shows that allow for electronic body scanning and clear information were already in our hands. So, certainty was always our goal, but unfortunately it was in many ways an illusion. We learned that where certainty leaves off, faith begins, and we found we were usually dealing with this blend. Life with cancer was rarely crystal clear.

Practice in Action

When faced with information, thoughts, or emotions, ask yourself whether they are factual, speculation, or imaginary and how they can benefit you or cause harm instead.

Beneficial Character Strengths

Discernment is perceiving and understanding oneself, others, and situations accurately and objectively, including discriminating between what is beneficial and what is harmful, without prejudice or bias.

— *Maximize Certainty* —

Patience is maintaining steady awareness and control of one's thoughts and responses while waiting for or seeking an outcome; controlling one's words and actions while willingly and calmly taking the time to respond to difficult, inconvenient, hurtful, delaying, or troublesome situations.

5 - Fact-Based Choice:
CHOOSE INTEGRATED TREATMENT

The Concept

Treatment choices for cancer are almost overwhelming in their range and complexity, especially for the more common types of the disease. However, not all treatments will be a fit for you. You and those helping with your care will benefit from exploring and understanding the applicable conventional medical, complementary, and alternative[1] treatments and their interactions and implications. Be cautious about feeling so desperate for a cure that you randomly try anything and everything that someone says might help. You could bankrupt your money, time, and energy in pursuing all options and opinions. On the other hand, you will also have to be courageous at times in trying options that you have never previously experienced or considered.

The goal is to integrate options in consultation with your doctor(s). In other words, you are responsible for creating

---

[1] "Complementary and Alternative Medicine (CAM) is a group of diverse medical and health care systems, practices, and products that are not presently considered to be part of conventional medicine. Complimentary medicine is used together with conventional medicine, and alternative medicine is used in place of conventional medicine. ... Defining CAM is difficult, because the field is very broad and constantly changing." For more detail on this topic, see **http://nccam.nih.gov/health/whatiscam**.

your own treatment plan in collaboration with your medical team, with the help of loved ones as needed, and adjusting it to changing circumstances. You then implement what is the best fit for you, keeping your doctors informed at all times and seeking their advice. Unfortunately, many doctors have limited training in and understanding of complementary and alternative treatments, so you may need to seek advisors beyond your geographical area. Because scientific evidence is limited about some alternative choices, you may choose an option that you personally find beneficial, as long as it doesn't interfere with or harm your conventional medical choices of treatment.

Personal Perspectives

Craig: I promised my doctors that I would keep them fully informed, and that I was choosing conventional treatment. However, I also investigated and tried many therapies beyond conventional medicine. I began with a message out to friends and family seeking well-researched conventional medicine treatments and well-researched alternative or complementary medicine and healing methods. I wanted the means of maintaining personal well-being and the strength of my body's immune system while undergoing the conventional medicine option. I was clear that I wanted to avoid receiving information about alternative approaches that were only anecdotally supported (for example, this worked for someone…). These, to me, bordered on pseudo-science, as they had no research demonstrating effectiveness.

I used hypnosis, acupuncture, homeopathy, ortho-bionomy, Reiki, Tai Chi, kinesiology, supplements, massage, nutrition, sea salt baths, music, art, visualization, and more. For supplements and nutrition choices, in particular, I consulted experts for the best choices for my particular type of cancer. I also carefully investigated potential interactions between my supplements and chemotherapy and radiation before proceeding and made adjustments as indicted. I investigated the issue of water quality and made the choice to drink filtered water and not drink from soft plastic containers. I believe the various therapies I used improved my quality of life and my longevity, because they improved my overall health, resilience, and strength.

Susanne: My role included providing the doctors with information about our choices and setting up alternative care appointments. However, my primary focus was on nutrition. I met with a doctor who specialized in cancer and diet, researched supplements and their potential interactions with drugs, and designed a diet that would work for both of us. I then did lots of cooking! I enjoyed successfully experimenting with ways to improve my husband's red blood cell counts by combining foods with vitamin C together with foods high in iron. The more normal his blood was, the better his energy level was. I was unable to find anything that increased the white blood cell count, but I was able to use nutrition and supplements to keep my husband's immune system protected, so he rarely became ill with conditions beyond cancer.

Practice in Action

Carefully investigate your options before choosing your treatment program. Be open to trying new foods prepared in new ways. Be very cautious about assuming something is safe or wise just because it is called or labeled "natural" or "organic".

Beneficial Character Strengths

Moderation is recognizing and avoiding extremes in use of time, words, actions, and other choices, to seek a balance that creates positive outcomes.

Courage is taking brave and bold action, defending what is right, or facing and completing a worthwhile challenge, even when experiencing fear, resistance, uncertainty, opposition, hardship, or possible danger.

6 - Fact-Based Choice 6: *CREATE A TEAM*

The Concept

While you may be tempted at times to isolate yourself, effectively responding to cancer requires a team approach. This means collaborating, cooperating, and consulting with helpful people and getting to know and trust the members of your doctors' teams. At times, you may have to insist that doctors and others talk to one another about your case, if it is not part of their normal routine. People are often specialists these days, and it is only through discussion that the broader picture and best view of your illness and health plan can emerge.

It can often be helpful to obtain second opinions and consult with experts about your potential choices. This can give you a level of comfort that everything possible is being done that can be done. This effort will be most effective if you have carefully tracked what has been done so far and also ask your medical institution to provide the consulting physician with complete records.

Depending on where you live and the resources in your community, you may be able to access and utilize support groups, counselors, and social workers. Many hospitals have social workers on staff who provide an empathetic listening ear, as well as referrals to trustworthy financial, legal, and community support resources. If you want to attend a support group and there is not one available at your hospital or in your community, you may be able to work with a social worker or doctor to start one. Alternatively, there are excellent cancer and caregiving support resources on the Internet.

It is also vital that you act as a team with your primary caregiver(s). If this is a close relative, such as a spouse, you may already have experiences of working together well. Responding to the illness may actually bring you closer together. However, providing care to someone during an illness is likely to strain even the best of relationships. Stress often magnifies tendencies towards anxiety, control, fear, and so on. If the two of you are having difficulties working together, you may need a counselor or social worker to help you.

The roles you or others play (paying bills, doing housework, driving…) may change to compensate for any impairment resulting from the disease or treatments. Resentment, anger, stress, and fatigue can all interfere in a smoothly working relationship. It is wise to stop and remember that you value the relationships with those helping you and strategize how to have both the relationship and the caregiving work well. Part of the solution may be delegating some caregiving tasks to others.

Personal Perspectives

Craig: My view was that having many team members was the best. I wanted a wide range of experts assisting me with healing, and a good support team as well. We built relationships with everyone from the administrative staff to the nurses and doctors, learning names and contact information as we went. I continued to stay in touch with what was happening in cancer treatment at other area medical facilities, so I then knew when to seek a second opinion.

When it was clear that my surgeon, oncologist, and radiation oncologist had differing views on test results or treatment plans, it was wise and helpful to have them talk together and involve me as needed. We came to better conclusions and action plans that way. I also asked that reports be copied to doctors who consulted on my case. The more informed everyone was, the better possible care I received.

I tried out resources such as support groups, and then assessed whether they were a fit for me. At times, a weekly cancer support group was helpful, and at times, it wasn't. Attending it became most helpful as my condition worsened. Many members attended for a while and then left during periods of remission. I consistently attended a monthly spiritual group at the cancer support center, however, and the members of it became a key part of my team.

Susanne: The nurses were wonderful in providing information, collaborating with the doctors, and spotting when we needed additional help. We especially found the social workers at the hospital and the cancer support center very helpful, compassionate listeners, who made excellent suggestions to help us with our situation or choices. Sometimes life felt very overwhelming, and they helped us step back and gain perspective. At times, they met with us as individuals, and at times they met with us together as a couple. Both were helpful.

Our team included doctors, nurses, and caregivers, but it definitely stretched beyond medical personnel as well. We needed to hire a trustworthy lawyer to re-do legal estate and property paperwork done by an unskilled lawyer. Bankers, financial advisors, life insurance agents, funeral directors, and more helped us through making the difficult decisions that faced us.

Practice in Action

Recognize that you are the team leader (or your caregiver is when you cannot be). Everyone else is a collaborator and partner with you.

Beneficial Character Strengths

Cooperation is working with others in harmony to create or accomplish something that would be more difficult or impossible to accomplish by one person working alone.

Trustworthiness is handling tasks, responsibilities, possessions, money, and information reliably and honestly, thereby earning the confidence of others.

7 - Fact-Based Choice:
IMPROVE THE PROCESS

The Concept

While you will do your best in the beginning to set up a team and treatment plan that works, you will likely be making choices under high-stress circumstances. You will learn from experience who are the helpful and useful members of your team and who are not, who is open to learning from you, and who is resistant to listening to you. Notice when you appreciate what someone does. Also notice when you become upset or angry about what a team member does or the way someone is doing something. Assess the skills and knowledge of all team members and their contributions to the healing process, and make adjustments as needed in what they are doing, their membership on your team, or the roles they play.

Be generous and sincere with your praise and appreciation for the wide range of people who are being of service to you. This tends to bring out the best in others and boosts your well-being. However, also recognize that when you are advocating for your life, it is not a time to resist making changes out of concern for hurting someone's feelings. High stress may be a factor in your resistance to making changes, but some of the stress you are feeling may be from having someone on your team who is not contributing the way you need them to.

In addition to assessing and improving your team, you can also have an attitude of openness and experimentation with other parts of your experience. You can use a creative spirit and help from others to address issues of your physical comfort, times of day to take medications, diet changes, and much more. Some of the choices in this book require stepping outside of your comfort zone and trying something new.

As you experience your cancer journey, you may note at times when something occurs systematically in your treatment environment that is actually counter-productive for optimum patient care. You can make suggestions for improvements in medical care or systems that will make the process better for you and for others.

Personal Perspectives

Craig: Each week before my radiation appointment, the nurse went through a set of questions to determine if any side effects were present. We reflected on how problem-oriented the questions were and that there were none to determine what positive state I was in or what was going well. The nurse and the radiation oncologist agreed to include a list of questions that we provided to add to her list:

1. Are you continuing your daily visualization to eliminate the cancer and treatment side effects? Yes/No; Is that working well? Yes/Somewhat/No
2. On a scale of 1-10, how do you rate your mental, emotional, and spiritual attitude and outlook?
3. On a scale of 1-10, how would you rate your overall feeling of well-being?
4. Compared to pre-tumor surgery, describe your activity level: the same, higher, less than
5. How many hours of employment did you successfully accomplish this past week?

One time we received a report of an MRI from one of our doctors before the rest of the medical team had reviewed it. The report was unhappy news; however, in the days that followed, the rest of the team felt there was an error in the test, and in fact, the news was not bad. We then requested a change in procedure that allowed time for team review of test results before they were given to us. This reduced the roller-coaster effect on our emotions.

After my tumor recurred, I decided to evaluate a completely new team and sought a second opinion. I was pleased with the meeting, but our pro-con list of factors that would have me make such a major change indicated that I was better staying with my current hospital and team.

When medical staff gave me exceptional service, I told them so and made a note of their names so we could let their supervisors know. When things did not go well, I also communicated the problems to someone who could do something about them, as much as possible with tactfulness and courtesy.

The instructions that came with my chemotherapy pills were to take them either one hour before or two hours after a meal. I learned through experimentation that my nausea was significantly reduced if I took the pills two hours after a high-protein meal. This turned out to be valuable information to share with the doctor as well, as it helped other patients.

Susanne: From the beginning of the cancer journey, we made the commitment to make a difference, something that was consistent with how we behaved before cancer! We felt that if we had to go through this difficulty, there had to be some positive outcomes from the experience. One of the ways that we accomplished this was to complete the evaluation forms that the hospitals sent to us, as well as answer their follow-up survey phone calls. I was often frustrated that the patient was surveyed and not the family, as I was often in a better position to observe quality of care than my husband was. When I had something important to say, therefore, I wrote a separate letter and included it with the patient's evaluation form. If a staff person was particularly helpful, we acknowledged them by name on the form. If there were systems and processes that needed to change, we were frank and honest about making suggestions.

Caregiving was a constant learning process. Making the bed differently, maintaining a safe environment, giving medications, cooking new foods, and more, all required me to be creative and flexible. As one small example, I tried using a small plastic container that had once held applesauce for my husband to use to take his pills. It was too big, and pills ended up on the floor. I then switched to coffee scoops, and they were just the right size.

Practice in Action

Pay attention to when something is not working well and creatively work for improvement.

Beneficial Character Strengths

Excellence is striving to achieve high standards and a superior quality of work and effort, as well as fulfilling one's potential for character growth and development.

Truthfulness is communicating accurately to convey one's best understanding of facts and feelings.

8 - Fact-Based Choice: *ASK FOR HELP*

The Concept

You may have learned to be very independent in your functioning as an adult. There may also be cultural or gender factors affecting your thinking that you should handle this "cancer problem" on your own. You may regard your illness as private and no one else's business. You will be most effective at healing, however, if you are kind and gentle with yourself, recognize your limitations, and ask for help as needed.

You may benefit from asking someone to be your partner in the healing process, whether a family member or friend. This person could accompany you on medical appointments, help you think of questions to ask the doctor, take notes, collect medical records, help with making medical decisions, and provide emotional support to you. As your condition changes, you may need more skilled caregivers and helpers. Be clear on what your needs are and also what is *not* helpful from others. If you don't already know, you will now learn which family members are effective on your team when directly involved, and which ones are not. You will often need others to help you with making good decisions, so carefully assess who should have access to your medical records and medical team members directly.

It is wise to listen carefully to the input and concerns of your caregivers and team members, both the words and the emotions behind the words. Often they have perspectives that are vital for you to consider. Personal empowerment includes having the strength and humility to also listen to and rely on others. You may not know what resources and people are available for your help unless you ask for assistance. Many facilities have social workers, nutritionists, physical/occupational therapists, and speech therapists to assist you with problems or care. As an example, you may unexpectedly spend longer in bed after a surgical procedure than anticipated and may benefit from requesting physical therapy to maintain muscle strength.

Personal Perspectives

Craig: My approach throughout was that I was determined to do whatever I could. I wanted to maintain my independence as much as possible, as well as continue contributing to my employer, community, and household. However, my surgery location was on the top of my head, so it was impossible for me to do wound care without help. At one point, I needed rides to work and could not travel for my job, so co-workers helped. I set up drivers to take me to daily radiation appointments, so my wife did not have to do all of them. As I went through further surgeries, I required rehabilitation assistance. As my cancer spread and I experienced seizures, my functionality decreased, and I required further help. I consistently expressed gratitude to those who helped me, and I did my best to have a positive attitude with them. This seemed to make it easier for people to help me when I needed it.

Due to hair loss, I wanted a hat that was better than the baseball cap or knit wool one that was the extent of my hat wardrobe. I asked for help in finding something that worked, and I settled on a brown beret. It was fun wearing it around, and I received many compliments on how good it looked on me and teasing about looking like a French artist.

Susanne: It's very difficult when looking after people and watching out for their safety and well-being to avoid slipping into the trap of doing everything for them. I often had to consciously step back and practice patience while my husband did things for himself. I learned to ask whether he wanted help or preferred doing a task for himself.

Most of our family lived out of town, so we fully used their help when they came to visit. Some tasks, such as helping with financial, legal, and other paperwork could be handled long-distance. Because our family resources were limited, we relied on community resources and friends extensively. I maintained ongoing to-do lists for helpers so that I could respond effectively when people offered to help. I had to remind myself regularly that others wanted to help and feel like they were contributing. This perspective assisted me with asking for help, instead of struggling with tasks and becoming exhausted or injured.

It was hard to significantly change my lifestyle to be a caregiver. I also had to take over many of the tasks that my husband was doing previously or find someone else to do them. It helped that my husband did not have an attitude of helplessness. Somehow, that made it easier to give help when it was needed. We were also blessed in the later stages with a relative who paid for a part-time caregiver so I did not become so exhausted.

Practice in Action

Whenever you think of something that needs to be done, ask yourself who else could do it, and request a specific person to carry out the task.

Beneficial Character Strengths

Helpfulness is taking appropriate action to address the needs or participate in solving the problems of others or oneself.

Humility is seeing the strengths, imperfections, abilities, accomplishments, failures, and all other aspects of oneself and others in realistic perspective; acting consistently according to principles, morals, and values rather than ego; and acknowledging the greatness of God.

9 - Fact-Based Choice: CHOOSE WHERE TO BE

The Concept

Throughout your cancer journey, you will likely be in a variety of settings. You may have to be in a hospital, rehabilitation facility, nursing home, or hospice center at times, and each one will require adjustments to new staff, different procedures, and a changed living area. You may also have to move to a different home or to a different place in your current home that is better set up to meet your needs or nearer to helpful resources. Being in new places is a creative opportunity to do your best to set up your environment in ways that help you to feel better and heal. It is also an opportunity to focus on using all the resources of a facility or your home to recover and maximize your healing.

As you live temporarily in new places, notice which ones are beneficial and which ones do not seem to promote your healing or well-being. Discuss those thoughts with your caregiver. You may also choose to travel to a treatment center and may have to adjust flexibly to new modes of transportation, a new culture, and perhaps a different language.

It is wise, however, to recognize when being at home is the best place for your well-being. Coping at home may require additional help or may feel scary at times, but a familiar environment can help you with relaxing and healing.

Personal Perspectives

Craig: At the beginning, I evaluated which hospital I wanted to be at for surgery and treatment and chose one. Each time I entered a new facility, I carried with me a photo of my wife and grandchildren. I also posted a visualization poster called "The Three Tools of Healing: Medical Treatment, Prayer, and Joy & Laughter". These consistent, positive images helped me to feel at home wherever I was. [See Appendix A for a copy of the poster.]

I traveled a few hundred miles to an integrative cancer treatment center one time. After that, I decided I would not do any further traveling to seek treatment. I still evaluated various programs offered in other states and countries, but I never saw anything that made me change my mind about my decision.

At one point, I was in a rehabilitation center for almost two months. Getting back home was wonderful! However, being home also brought new challenges. I often had to sleep in a separate bed or area away from my wife, and we had to constantly rearrange our home to accommodate my changing physical condition and medical support equipment. In my new bedroom, I had family members hang photos and posters on the wall to encourage and inspire me.

Susanne: When my husband went through a rehabilitation program, I took photos of the obstacles and challenges of our home and brought them in for the therapy staff to evaluate. This helped them realize that my husband needed a different type of brace on his leg and that they needed to have him well enough to walk with a cane instead of relying on a walker. We made many modifications to our home to accommodate the needed changes, particularly safety bars. These turned out to be beneficial for guests and me as well!

We also had occupational and physical therapists come into our home to teach us what we needed to know. They identified when we needed a wheelchair ramp. They helped us learn about moving around our home safely, effective ways to get in and out of the shower, how to get clothes on and off more easily, and how to have my husband keep doing the dishes from his wheelchair, something I appreciated very much. Their education helped raise my confidence level significantly.

I was relieved at my husband's decision to minimize travel, which was exhausting to manage, but I would have done it if I had to. Every time that my husband came home after an extended absence in a hospital or care facility, there were new challenges to handle, so I was often scared about whether I could take care of him well at home. Friends and our support team encouraged me as needed. Home did consistently turn out to be the best place for him.

Practice in Action

Choose which items from home are the most beneficial and comforting for you to have with you when you have to stay away from home or in a new part of your home.

Beneficial Character Strengths

Flexibility is adjusting to life as it happens and embracing changes as needed, while remaining true to one's core values, beliefs, and appropriate priorities.

Resilience is accepting, responding appropriately to, recovering from, and coping with adversity, misfortune, change, or illness, and bouncing back from stressful experiences effectively and in a reasonable amount of time.

10 - Fact-Based Choice: COMMUNICATE WELL

The Concept

Communication opens up realistic new possibilities for your healing and well-being. You are responsible for promptly informing your caregivers and your medical team about any symptoms or side effects you are experiencing so they can respond effectively. They are handicapped in helping you if you do not provide them with clear facts, so it is important to commit to sharing. This shows respect for yourself and your well-being, as well as for those helping you. At times, you may need to delegate communications to your caregiver or accept feedback from your caregiver that you are having difficulty communicating well to the doctor. Unfortunately, one of the outcomes of cancer and its treatments can be impairment in thinking processes and speaking clearly.

Effectively and completely answer the questions of your medical team as best as you can, but don't wait to be asked how you are feeling when you are aware that something has changed. When you clearly communicate to your medical and care team, as well as with relatives and friends, you can then draw on their collective knowledge, experience, and wisdom. Be aware when your doctors may be distracted or rushed and help them to pause and listen when you have something important to say.

— Communicate Well —

As you assess the facts of your circumstances, it may also become clear to you that others may need whatever information you learn or discover on your journey. Remember that no matter how well informed a doctor is, cancer care, research, and treatments are changing globally on a daily basis. Do not assume that your doctor knows about all of the information you find, and share it. As you and your doctors find new options for treatment, discuss them and decide whether to make new choices. Know the variety of ways to communicate to your doctors, such as by phone, e-mail, or fax, as well as the ways they prefer to receive communications. You do not ever have to wait for a scheduled appointment to raise a concern, as action on your part could result in addressing an issue before it is a large problem.

Fellow support group members or other cancer patients can benefit from what you learn. It can be helpful to create email communications, a blog, documents, or reports for your own use and to help your medical and care providers, as well as your family and friends. These communications will help everyone who needs to know about you better understand what you are doing and why you are making your choices.

Personal Perspectives

Craig: My norm before cancer was to wait to report symptoms until I figured out whether they were serious. I learned quickly while dealing with cancer that waiting to report how I was doing handicapped my caregiver and my doctors. The earlier we had a warning that something might be changing, the better everyone responded, and the healthier I stayed.

Early in my cancer journey, I established a blog to share what was happening [www.factbasedspiritguidedpath.blogspot.com]. I felt empowered being in charge of communicating my new insights with people. I quickly learned, however, that medications and the cancer sometimes skewed my judgment about what I was saying, so I agreed with my wife that she would review my writing before I posted it. This turned into a rich blessing, as she often reminded me to share something that I'd forgotten, and she began to add her own comments under the heading of "the rest of the story"!

Susanne: I was very frank with my husband about reporting symptoms...that I wasn't able to be effective as his caregiver unless he was honest and prompt with telling me what I needed to know. Together we took our business and computer skills and developed spreadsheets to help us. We tracked my husband's symptoms against the possible side effects listed for the chemotherapy. We set up a chart of the regular blood test results so we knew what the normal results should be, where he was instead, and the trends. Tracking this information helped me make diet adjustments or request the doctor to consider a transfusion. Most helpful was the spreadsheet we did for medications and dosages (see sample below). Not only did my husband and I need to know what medications to dispense and when he should take them, but everyone else wanted to know this information, too. With the list computerized, we could easily print copies out for nurses, doctors, radiology staff, physical and occupational therapists, hospice workers, and more.

Date Started	Ordered By	Type/Names	Breakfast	Lunch	Dinner	Bedtime	Purpose
		Prescriptions and Over-the-Counter Pills					
		Supplements and Vitamins					
		TOTAL PER MEAL					

Practice in Action

During crisis management, over-communicate and don't make assumptions about what is important and what isn't. During calm periods, stay in communication about anything that changes or when you have questions or concerns.

Beneficial Character Strengths

Honesty is acting and speaking consistently with high and incorruptible moral, ethical, and legal standards.

Respect is interacting with all people and what they value, as well as animals and the environment, in a manner that demonstrates they are worthy of fair treatment, consideration, and honorable regard.

Part 2: The Spirit-Guided Choices

Note: The Spirit-Guided Choices here in Part 2 are ideally *integrated* in action with Part 1, the Fact-Based Choices.

1 - Spirit-Guided Choice: ENGAGE IN PRAYER

The Concept

You may or may not be comfortable with the idea of praying for healing, help, and guidance. If you quiet yourself, however, you may notice that there is a natural impulse within you to reach out to something or Someone for aid and comfort. Alternatively, prayer may already be a part of your daily life, and the diagnosis of cancer simply has you increasing the amount you are praying. Prayers may be in a published book or simple words from your heart. Prayer helps bring a sense of peace in the middle of chaos and increases the love and compassion you feel for yourself and for those traveling this cancer journey with you.

Essentially, you will find it more empowering responding to something as big as cancer by drawing on spiritual strength. When the plain facts are inadequate, when you are in pain or despair, when you don't know what choices to make, prayer can provide nourishment, comfort, and answers. Just remember that an answer to prayers is not always "yes" or exactly what you ask to happen. Sometimes the answer may be "no" or "please wait."

When considering including prayer as one of your healing choices, you can take the perspective that all true healing comes from God. This then says that you and the medical staff have to do the footwork, but in the greater perspective, how much healing happens is out of your hands. Be aware of your medical staff's attitude towards spirituality and prayer. They may also be willing to pray with or for you.

In addition to praying for healing for yourself, you can request that others pray in person or over the phone or Internet with you. You can also pray for those caring for you, that they have the needed knowledge, skill, strength, and well-being to assist you. In addition, you can increase your empowerment by requesting prayers from others as needed and appropriate. Group worship of some form may also strengthen you spiritually.

Personal Perspectives

Craig: Throughout my adult life, I recall having had an ongoing hunger for really connecting with prayer at a depth at which I could honestly say my soul was touched and renewed. There were fleeting moments, but there was nothing sustainable. As I began responding to my cancer diagnosis, I significantly increased my connection to God. I was much more comfortable dealing with the facts and situations filled with certainty. It was a real challenge for me to face uncertainty, and prayer helped me deal with that.

During the first week after the tumor was discovered, I lived in a continual state of prayer. Later, faced with the terror of possible tumor re-growth, spiritual tools helped me to feel empowered to respond with defining options and paths to choose. Whenever I needed to make new treatment choices, I learned the facts, consulted with those I needed input from, and then turned to prayer for guidance and confirmation of the best choice. Actually, I found it beneficial throughout my cancer journey to draw on prayer.

Susanne: Sometimes my prayers were constant, but at other times, they didn't go beyond "O God, help!". Sometimes I was so exhausted and overwhelmed that I even had to delegate the praying to others! We tried our best to continue having couple prayer time, even when hospitalizations intervened. We made the commitment to host a regular spiritual study circle in our home and keep it going except when hospitalizations made it impossible. The participants turned into wonderful friends and became our prayer partners, cheerleaders, and supporters as we explored such topics together as making spiritual choices, prayer, the life of the soul, and life after death.

Practice in Action

Say, "O God, I need Your help!" when difficult news or events come, rather than swearing.

Beneficial Character Strengths

Compassion is feeling genuine concern for others and oneself, empathizing with the pain and suffering of those in difficult situations, and seeking ways to relieve their pain and ease their suffering.

Spirituality is nurturing your heart and soul through maintaining a close, interactive relationship with God, drawing on spiritual sources for divine guidance, dedicated or devoted to the service of God or religion, and acting and speaking in alignment with the teachings in the Word of God.

2 - Spirit-Guided Choices: MEDITATE AND VISUALIZE

The Concept
Meditation is a reflective process that allows you to calmly center yourself and be open to peace, healing, and answers. The intention is to detach from what is happening around you and the need to be in control of it, and then quieting the activity of the mind. When you become aware of your quieter, inner thoughts, then spiritual insights and guidance can emerge. There are many methods, so you can choose whichever one(s) you are comfortable using.

While you may simply meditate to lower your anxiety level or focus on inner healing, you can also use it to focus on practical matters. You have the opportunity to listen to and respect your intuition about choices to make. You can use meditation to reflect on how to respond to the illness and to receive answers to questions that you pose to yourself. For instance, you might meditate on when to start or stop treatments, how to resolve an issue with a friend, or whether to keep working or take a leave of absence.

Visualization is a tool that involves picturing yourself in a particular situation, and also creating a mental image of you doing whatever is called for in that situation. While doing the visualizing, focus on generating the feelings you want to experience there. This practice can help you create a mindset for healing and help you reduce your fears about what is happening or what might happen in the future. Alternatively, you can reduce your stress level by visualizing yourself in nature or some other beautiful environment while focusing on breathing deeply and relaxing.

Visualizing your goals can also help you with achieving them. You can picture being healthy, peaceful, in action, accepting, hopeful, relaxed, of effective service to others, or whatever state you desire. When you have a clear vision of what you want to achieve, this empowers you to actually achieve these outcomes. There are many visualization media that you can purchase as CD's, DVD's, or Internet downloads, but you can also create your own, perhaps with the help of others. [We found ones by Dr. Bernie Siegel and Belleruth Naparstek particularly helpful.]

Personal Perspectives
Craig: I carried, posted in my hospital rooms, and shared hundreds of copies of a beautiful poster entitled "The Three Tools of Healing: Medical Treatment, Prayer, and Joy & Laughter." [See Appendix A for a copy of the poster.] It gave me a regular focus for meditation and visualization. In addition, I often found it helpful to involve others in creating visualizations for me or meditating with me. Before my first tumor removal surgery, I visualized creating a cocoon around the tumor so that the doctors could remove it in one piece. A friend helped me to verbalize and release my fear that the surgeon might not be able to fully remove my tumor. This friend then helped me to visualize sealing every crack and crevice in the capsule around the tumor with SuperGlue®...no using duct tape, which I loved to use in repair projects! The tumor actually and unusually came out in one solid piece.

When it was time for me to receive radiation and chemotherapy, I took markers and paper and drew a vision of my healing. The drawing of myself showed my treatment, my dis-

— *Meditate and Visualize* —

ease, and my white blood cells eliminating the disease. I drew a side view of my head showing the location where the tumor was removed. I depicted the last little pieces of the tumor as red squiggly lines and outlined my plan as follows:

- Engage in prayer, meditation, and visualization to support the white blood cells in creating a barrier around any pieces of the tumor that may have infiltrated the brain beyond the solid tumor. Invite the tumor cells to entirely leave my body. Visualize minimizing or eliminating any potential side effects of the radiation and chemotherapy.
- Continue to eat good food, take supplements, and participate in exercise to keep me strong and healthy, and to minimize or eliminate the side effects of the radiation and chemotherapy.
- Welcome radiation and chemotherapy to neutralize the tumor pieces, so they can be carried away by the white blood cells.
- Hold as my goal effective and efficient healing with long-term survival and excellent quality of life.

I had another friend create a visualization for me after treatment ended that would keep me focused on healing. I recorded it and put it on my MP3 player, so I could listen to it regularly.

Susanne: I found as caregiver that I was always in motion, and when I was not in motion, my mind was thinking of what there was to do. Sitting and calmly meditating on my own was very difficult. However, I did use a visualization CD when I needed to calm my mind and rest or sleep. It mentally placed me in beautiful places out in nature, which are generally happy, healing places for me to be. On respite days, I usually spent time out in nature or in quiet places that allowed me to re-center myself. I also found it helpful to occasionally attend or host group meditation sessions led by friends of ours.

Practice in Action

When your thoughts are racing or whirling, deep, regular breathing and focusing on something beautiful can calm and center you. It can be helpful to choose and say a specific affirmation statement as well, such as:
- I am strong, healthy, and making wise choices.
- I have the resources I need to be healthy.
- I am happy and peaceful at this moment.

Beneficial Character Strengths

Beauty is expressing the best of one's inner spirit and demonstrating, seeing, and creating attractiveness, loveliness, or order wherever possible.

Detachment is stepping back to gain a different perspective on what is happening and placing less importance on worldly concerns, while selflessly letting go of one's feelings, hopes, desires, attachments, and need to be in control.

3 - Spirit-Guided Choice:
SEEK INSPIRATION

The Concept

It takes significant effort to travel the cancer journey and hold onto hope for a cure or for quality of life while you are ill or healing. You need to feel supported in your effort to keep going. However, it may take some exploration to find what inspires, encourages, uplifts, and heals you. Some possibilities are stories, poems, articles, books, faith-based materials, movies, video clips, photographs, posters, time out in nature, and music. It can be especially helpful to hear the stories of those who are surviving the experience of cancer or to receive encouraging messages from family, friends, and medical staff. Be conscious of when you need to have something inspirational with you, such as during inpatient stays and while waiting for difficult outpatient medical appointments.

There are times during medical tests and treatments when you can include your own inspirational music. MRI and radiation technicians will often agree to play your own CD, and devices such as MP3 players may be allowed for some surgeries. Music can carry you mentally and emotionally away from difficult experiences and help you better cope with them. Inspirational music can also encourage you to focus on healing.

Personal Perspectives

Craig: When I found positive and inspiring material that gave me hope, I passed it along to my family and friends to lift their spirits as well. At one point, I was inspired with a new image of how I was seeing my journey as a bird in flight:
    a. The body of the bird was the medical treatment.
    b. One wing was prayer, meditation, and visualization.
    c. The other wing was nutrition, supplements, and exercise.
    d. Joy and laughter created an uplift of wind under the wings.

It raised my spirits each time I envisioned this image!

Susanne: My biggest inspiration was watching my husband expand his spirituality and handle the cancer journey with such grace and strength. Beyond that, however, I drew on scripture, spiritual study groups, books, framed quotations, music, and time outdoors. Usually whenever I felt low, something inspirational would occur that lifted me up and kept me going. Often what I received was encouraging notes from friends and family.

Some days I felt as if I was living out my life in doctor's waiting rooms (or having scary moments like seeing my husband strapped to a radiation table in a mask!). Hospitals, in particular, seem to suck the life out of people…me and everyone else. This is so strange when they are supposed to be a healing environment. Appointments often interfered with normal meal schedules, and people took us into enclosed boxes of rooms with no access to sunlight or nature…anything to suggest life. We consciously made the effort to seek out plants and flowers, artwork, or non-medical corners of these facilities to provide some balance.

— Seek Inspiration —

Practice in Action

Keep inspirational material in various places in your life—bedside table, living room, kitchen, car, briefcase, purse, or jacket pocket—so you always have something uplifting nearby.

Beneficial Character Strengths

Encouragement is offering sincere, uplifting acknowledgment of the character strengths, effective actions, or good intentions of others and oneself; inspiring or assisting others and oneself to start, continue, or stop doing something; and fostering personal growth and development.

Joyfulness is being in a state of high-spirited and ecstatic delight, gladness, blissfulness, great happiness, and jubilation.

4 - Spirit-Guided Choice: EXPERIENCE THE ARTS

The Concept

We have left and right brains that provide balance in our lives. Often one side of the brain is dominant, however. If you are more "left-brained," you tend to approach life logically and in a linear, straightforward fashion, often relying on numbers to quantify matters. If you are more "right-brained," you tend to be more creative and flexible in your approach. Creative arts tend to draw on the right side of the brain and assist people with emotional expression.

Experiencing cancer causes a variety of emotions to arise, and it can be difficult to understand them and express them appropriately. Working with your hands in some way and the arts are outlets for your thoughts and feelings, and they can help you with healing emotionally, mentally, spiritually, and physically. They have the power to transform your thoughts, feelings, outlooks, spirits, and actions.

"The arts" is actually a very broad term, so there are many opportunities to connect with them. People often have a tendency to say things like, "I'm not artistic" or "I'm not good at XX." At this point in your life, what do you have to lose by trying something new? The following lists of art possibilities are not complete, but they likely contain some that you have not yet considered doing. You can experiment with whatever benefits you. Remember that incorporating the arts into your healing journey is sometimes "doing" the art and sometimes participating by "observing," such as visiting an art museum or watching a performance.

Examples of Arts and Crafts Activities
- Performing Arts
- Attending events
- Making/Listening to music
- Acting
- Directing
- Producing
- Dancing
- Singing
- Visual Arts
- Movies, videos, and slide presentations
- Architecture
- Photography
- Animation and computer graphics
- Painting - multiple media
- Drawing
- Gardening
- Crafts
- Weaving
- Pottery
- Sculpture
- Clothing design; Sewing
- Embroidery
- Knitting and crocheting
- Ceramics
- Jewelry-making
- Furniture-making
- Leatherwork
- Basket-weaving
- Glassblowing

- Candle-making
- Print-making
- Puppet-making
- Toy-making
- Calligraphy
- Hair design
- Tattoos
- Flower arranging

Reading and Writing Arts
- Dramatic reading
- Story writing
- Storytelling
- Scriptwriting
- Book writing
- Poetry writing
- Journal writing

Social Arts
- Welcoming
- Introductions and remembering names
- Conversation
- Cooking and food preparation
- Hospitality/Serving
- Creating ceremonies

Personal Perspectives

Craig: Occasionally I wrote poetry, but my strongest connection to engaging in the arts came once hospice services began. We had both an art therapist and a music therapist. The art therapist helped my wife and I both paint how we were feeling about what was happening. She left paints at our home, and I continued to paint regularly between visits.

The music therapist helped me to continue singing my favorite prayers and songs, even when communication became difficult for me. She took two poems that I wrote many years ago and composed music for them and helped me sing them. My wife and I compiled the story of my life illustrated by my poetry, prose, and artwork from throughout the years as well as from the time since the cancer diagnosis. We also gathered and made recordings of my singing. All of these experiences brought me great joy.

Susanne: I've been a writer for many years, so it was actually painful to lose much of my writing time while doing caregiving. Adding comments to the blog my husband began, and later writing it entirely, gave me a consistent and helpful outlet for sharing about our experiences. Music was consistently uplifting for me. One of the most significant blessings of the hospice period, and in fact of our marriage, was the artistic expression that arose in the last months of my husband's life. It was a joy to watch him paint, and it was a privilege to put together a book portraying the story of his life's transformation.

Practice in Action

Keep supplies on hand, such as colored markers or musical recordings, and look for opportunities to attend events that nourish your soul or stimulate your creativity.

Beneficial Character Strengths

Confidence is trusting one's inner value, worthy intentions, capacity to think and act effectively, and ability to accomplish stated goals of oneself and of others.

Creativity is drawing on ideas, inspiration, or imagination to develop or produce something new, including contributions and solutions that benefit others.

5 - Spirit-Guided Choice:
STRIVE TO BE YOUR BEST

The Concept

This choice is based on the philosophy that life is a learning adventure that provides you with endless opportunities to improve how you speak and act, and to strive for excellence. If you look for lessons in your cancer-related experiences that help your personal growth, it will provide meaning to them. The purpose of engaging in continuous improvement of your mind, heart, and character is inner peacefulness, better relationships, and skills that you may need in the future.

It can be easy in the middle of dealing with cancer to think that everyone should simply be compassionate and accommodate your bad moods, difficult attitudes, and hurtful words and actions. However, this is abdicating your personal responsibility and power. This illness is a test that may be uniquely suited to helping you overcome character faults that have troubled you and your relationships much of your life. Your experiences with cancer and treatments can also help you develop new strengths.

Striving to be your best requires you to mindfully assess how you speak and act in every situation that occurs, whether at home, work, the community, or in your medical treatment environment. In every moment, you can choose the "higher" path or the "lower" one. You can apply character qualities appropriately to situations, such as *assertiveness, compassion, patience*, *resilience*, or *wisdom*. You can be *friendly*, *courteous*, and *considerate* with each person you interact with during the healing process. You can show *trust* and *confidence* in and appreciation for the medical and support team you create. In addition, you can practice *flexibility* when faced with the constantly changing "new normal" that becomes part of living with cancer, its treatments, and its outcomes.

The more you are able to be courteous to medical staff, the easier it will be for them to give you the best care. Unfortunately, disease, medications, and treatments can change people's personality and at times destroy the controls that people normally have on their speech and actions. Outwardly being your best in this circumstance can be virtually impossible. Your family may then be able to assist medical personnel and caregivers to be compassionate towards you, or social workers or medical staff may help family members do the same.

Personal Perspectives

Craig: I had to be constantly flexible, as both my treatment plan and where I had to be for medical care kept changing. Overall, I did my best to be friendly and easy to work with for the staff wherever I was, only occasionally getting frustrated with people, and I appreciated the same attitudes from them.

Practicing patience has been a life-long challenge, and as I lost functionality and depended more and more on others, I had to strengthen this quality. It was close to impossible to practice patience when I was losing the ability to speak, however. Sometimes the frustration of understanding but not being able to express myself was almost more than I could bear.

Susanne: Shortly after my husband's tumor diagnosis, I recognized that this challenge was an opportunity for me to strengthen the qualities of humility and detachment. Repeatedly, I had to humbly recognize that I didn't have all the answers or the control over whether my husband lived or died. I had to detach from knowing what the future held for both of us and from being so emotionally tied to my husband that I couldn't picture living without him. Often I felt humbled by watching the loving way my husband interacted with others, even when he was in the midst of very difficult experiences. He was often my power of example. Flexibility became vital for me to practice as well. Nothing stayed the same for very long.

Practice in Action

Choose one or two character qualities that you want to strengthen and set specific goals and action plans to improve them. (See Appendix B for ideas.)

Beneficial Character Strengths

Excellence is striving to achieve high standards and a superior quality of work and effort, as well as fulfilling one's potential for character growth and development.

Perseverance is persisting and pressing onward towards worthwhile goals, particularly in the face of challenges or adversity.

6 - Spirit-Guided Choice:
SERVE OTHERS

The Concept

One of life's wisdoms is that when we strive to lighten the difficulties of others, we lighten our own burdens. The more we focus on our own selves, and particularly when we mire ourselves in self-pity and complaints, the more miserable we feel. Service to others is a vital component of living a spiritual life. It is acting selflessly or sacrificially to improve or enhance the welfare and quality of life of others and their situations and experiences. It calls you to consciously observe and reflect on how to make a positive difference for others and then step into effective action to carry it out. Often those you serve will be your fellow cancer patients or your caregivers.

Service can vary from large civic projects down to brief acts that have an effect on others. You could send someone a card, pull a weed from the garden, or simply offer a genuine smile to another. The size of the act is not the point; lifting the hearts of others is the goal. You will find your own happiness increases in response. When you don't feel well, serving others may seem like the last thing you want to do. Perhaps in that moment, the service you offer is softening your voice so that your caregiver finds your complaints less difficult to hear.

Service connects you with love to others. In your love for other human beings, you look to make their lives easier. You seek ways to contribute to them in some way. Serving others creates emotional and spiritual healing for you and for them.

Personal Perspectives

Craig: Being of service to others has been part of my life as long as I can remember. As I went through the cancer experience, I consciously looked for what to say to help staff members and fellow support group members. I had conversations with them about relationships, their spiritual paths, and more. I also shared my own experiences. I looked for helpful articles, books, or other materials that would ease others' difficulties. Sometimes the biggest service I could give was being cooperative with the care others gave to me.

As my cancer journey advanced, I began to look at the legacy that I wanted to leave that would continue to serve others. This included financial gifts and arrangements, cards and notes for people, and creative projects. My wife helped me leave a message for my daughter's wedding day and birthday cards for family members.

Susanne: Caregiving is a full-time service project. For me to be effective at it, I analyzed my husband's needs every step of the way, usually in consultation with him and his medical team. My goal was always his comfort and happiness. At one point, though, I noticed that while my service to my husband was primarily out of love, there was also a key element of fear—if I didn't take good care of him, bad things would happen to one or both of us. It took regular prayer to shrink this fear to manageable size and hold onto faith instead.

One of the many things that made caregiving easier was that my husband regularly expressed appreciation. I knew that he was grateful for what I was doing for him, even when the whole grain organic bread I served him tasted like thin cardboard! When I struggled with fatigue, anger, or whether I could keep going, I set up a respite day or arranged for extra help. This allowed me to breathe, rest, and re-focus. I could let go of any anger or resentment I was starting to feel and rebalance into feeling loving.

Practice in Action

Set a goal each day to find some new way to be of service to someone, no matter how small the action.

Beneficial Character Strengths

Cooperation is working with others in harmony to create or accomplish something that would be more difficult or impossible to accomplish by one person working alone.

Thoughtfulness is being concerned in a deliberate and genuine way about the well-being and happiness of others, acting in anticipation of and in loving awareness of their needs.

7 - Spirit-Guided Choice: *BUILD UNITY*

The Concept

Throughout our lives, we speak and act in ways that sometimes result in tasks, projects, or relationships that are "incomplete." They are unfinished or have outstanding issues. These "incompletions" may weigh on your mind and heart or be troubling to others. Serious illness and the prospect of dying are a wake-up call that time is limited, and leaving important matters unattended is unwise. As much as possible taking action to complete what is undone is a key part of your healing process.

Everything from organizing family paperwork to forgiving your best friend or a parent can help you to heal. Reconciling estrangements between you and others, in particular, can help your healing process. Building unity with others creates strength in you and expands your support team. Facing major illness can provide opportunities for you and others to re-evaluate the quality of the relationship you have together, and where applicable, express remorse, apologize, and forgive. It is wise to recognize that you may not be able to do many completion or unity-building actions without assistance from others. You may need to ask for help. For instance, your doctor may be able to refer you to a helpful social worker, support group, or counselor.

The medical community is not perfect, and people on your team may make mistakes in your care. They are often then constrained in being accountable and apologizing for their mistakes out of fear of legal action or retribution against them. It is wise for you to be aware if you are feeling resentment or anger towards someone on your team. You may be able to resolve the issue with that person directly or seek assistance from someone else on the staff. You may also have to accept, forgive, and move forward.

Unity is consciously looking for and strengthening points of commonality, harmony, and attraction, as well as working with others to build a strong foundation of oneness, love, commitment, and cooperation. Creating unity between people releases positive, loving energy into your healing environment. Life is short for everyone…it's not worth spending it holding onto grudges or resentments and being stubborn about who should reach out first. Building unity can occur through communicating more often, sharing time together with others, letting the little things go, and looking for points of agreement with others.

Personal Perspectives

Craig: I had made great progress over the years in re-establishing strong relationships with my family. My relationship with my adult son, however, was still very poor at the time of my diagnosis. He was also diagnosed with a brain tumor four months before me at the exact time his son was born, and he was experiencing cancer treatment. I felt as if I just wanted to hold him in my arms and protect and cherish him, but I had no idea how to do it. How could I overcome the past deficit in our relationship? The miracle was that our shared walk along the cancer path helped us to heal our estrangement and find peace and love with one another. In addition to my asking him to forgive me for my mistakes of the past, we began to have more frequent lunches out together and increased our phone calls to one another.

Susanne: Initially when my husband became ill, I found it difficult raising issues with him. It seemed wrong somehow to be upset or angry about something he did when I wasn't experiencing something as big as cancer. However, we needed to behave like a normal couple and address issues that arose. Sometimes I talked problems through with a friend first or used a journal to clarify my thoughts and emotions. I determined it was more loving and peaceful in our relationship if we simply kept things "cleaned up" along the way.

We did our best to stay consistent with having "dates" out with each other. When going out became difficult, we would sit and watch a movie together or play a board or card game at home. We kept our practice in place of praying together, which helped us find a calm, connected space each day. As it became difficult to sleep with one another due to my husband's physical challenges, we got creative with occasionally sharing his single hospital bed or using a separate fold-out bed near his room for "double-bed time."

I was more likely to observe and become upset over errors on the part of medical staff than my husband was. Because we were using a teaching hospital, I often chose to simply inform someone of the error. I encouraged the feedback to be used as a learning opportunity, making it clear that I was not seeking legal action or looking for resolution or action beyond education.

Practice in Action

Notice when you have an uncomfortable feeling somewhere in your body; such as tightness in your chest, held breath, or a tense or upset stomach that is not illness or drug related. Assess whether these symptoms relate to unhappiness or anger about a relationship, or fear and grief with circumstances, and take steps to find solutions.

Beneficial Character Strengths

Forgiveness is pardoning someone for saying or doing something hurtful or harmful, giving up a desire for revenge, and letting go of anger and resentment.

Responsibility is claiming personal accountability for one's own life, choices, happiness, commitments, required activities, and relationships with others, as well as sharing accountability for the quality of life in the communities in which one lives and works and the global society.

8 - Spirit-Guided Choice: *EXPAND LOVE*

The Concept

Love is a powerful force for healing and happiness. The more that you generate, express, and expand the loving feelings that you have for your family and friends, the easier your cancer journey is likely to be. The more you are aware of how love can spread through your words and actions to everyone around you, the more love you will generate and receive. If you are having times of feeling unloving towards others, increasing your loving words and actions will likely help release true feelings of love towards them.

One of the wisdoms in life is that negative emotions and atmospheres seem to promote illness or unbalance in us. Positive ones seem to create more opportunity for health and wellbeing. It is infinitely easier for others to be willing to help you, and help you more effectively, when you are loving with them rather than cranky or mean!

You may also be wise to pay attention to whether you are feeling loving towards yourself. Are you blaming yourself for this illness? Are you criticizing yourself continually for words you spoke or actions you took? Are you resenting that you can no longer do things instead of feeling grateful for what you can do and the loving help others are giving to you? Instead, are you taking good care of yourself and practicing self-forgiveness? Are you being kind and gentle to yourself during this difficult time?

Sometimes you may think that love should be limited to a few close people. However, the power of love is broad enough to include everyone. It can be stress relieving and loving to allow others to accompany you and your family on this journey. Being loving even to those you don't know, including medical and caregiving staff, generates a positive force within you that helps with your healing.

It is also wise to spend time feeling connected to the Universal Love that comes from God (see Choice 1, Engage in Prayer). Receiving Divine Love may be all that sustains you at some of the most difficult moments, and it can soften the rawness of your experiences.

Personal Perspectives

Craig: I lost track of the stream of people who called and visited me, because there were so many. I felt surrounded by love, and my spirit was uplifted. I think visiting me touched others' hearts, too. I got a call late one night from a dear friend who is the crusty outside/heart-of-gold inside type. He said to me "Sorry I didn't call sooner, but I'm not real good at this sympathy and condolence stuff." I said, "I don't need that stuff!!! I need your good wishes, your prayers, and for you to be happy! Can you get on board with that???" That shifted the conversation real quick.

Often when I was in the hospital, attending support group meetings, or going to medical appointments, I wore an "I Love My Wife" button. She normally wore her corresponding "I Love My Husband" button, too. We felt it was helpful to continually affirm our love for one another and our support of each other in this way. It also helped staff with remembering us, something that can be difficult in large medical institutions.

Susanne: I made the commitment early on with my husband's illness that I would communicate to others what we were going through and request their prayers, visits, food, flowers, cards, or whatever else we needed from them. I also tried to communicate when we had any limitations of time and energy for them to respect. We then received "love notes", emails, and cards from friends locally and from around the planet regularly. Often the communications came at low moments when we needed the love and uplifting thoughts.

Friends and family often spent time at our home as well, bringing a meal, helping with household organization and tasks, sorting out finances, or doing home maintenance. Sometimes they simply sat with us, listening and accompanying us. It was such a relief to feel their love and know that we were not alone. On the other hand, I needed quiet time to rebuild my energy, and the constant socializing was a strain at times.

Although we had a strong marriage prior to the cancer diagnosis, we still had times of feeling disconnected from each other due to disruptions in our routines, medical procedures, and endless fatigue. It helped us to regularly say, "I love you," far more than we had in the past. Saying prayers together also helped us to regenerate feeling connected with one another.

Practice in Action
Say "I love you" whenever possible to family members and friends.

Beneficial Character Strengths
Friendliness is demonstrating an outgoing and positive social attitude and reaching out to connect with and build relationships with people.

— *Expand Love* —

Love is connecting to others through affection and joining with them to express the powerfully magnetic and caring force that unites the universe.

9 - Spirit-Guided Choice: FEEL HAPPY

The Concept

You likely have a mental list of what makes you feel happy, and it's probably different from the lists of others close to you. Happiness is often connected to what is going well in life. It takes an extraordinary effort at times to feel happy while dealing with devastating illnesses such as cancer. However, it is possible to have happy thoughts, even if it is only for a few minutes of each day. You will notice that there can even be long stretches of time when your illness is not on your mind and you can focus on pure enjoyment of where you are, what you are doing, and whom you are with. If you are positive in your attitude, it will make it easier for your medical team and caregivers to also be upbeat with you.

In the past, you may have taken your happy and contented moments for granted. Now it's wise to consciously determine what you will do to uplift your spirits and include it in your life. Notice that you can engage in what creates joy, laughter, and fun, even if it is simply making jokes about weird or awful things that are happening. Joyfulness increases your strength and helps you think more clearly. It is easier to cope with all the changes and challenges in your life. As much as possible, engage in the activities that you have always enjoyed, even if it means making accommodation for temporary or permanent impairments.

When there is a mix of happy and sad events happening, it can be helpful to practice identifying what you are thankful for in your life. Practicing gratitude can often lift your spirits.

Personal Perspectives

Craig: My positive attitude helped me strengthen my health and lengthen my life. I particularly felt very, very happy to feel spiritually transformed in the process of dealing with cancer. I felt really connected in my prayers and meditation in a way that had never happened in my life before. My biggest unhappiness was the continual increase in my physical limitations, although each time I successfully accomplished an improvement was grounds to feel happy. I was happy when I could drive, work, do household maintenance, or whatever seemed "normal." It made me happy when I saw my wife having "normal" moments, too, like getting to the pool to swim or working part-time.

We initially had a practice of daily listing what we were grateful for. However, we shifted the practice after a discussion at a cancer spirituality group meeting. We still shared gratitude for the "roses"—the good that was happening in our lives. However, we began to list the "thorns" of the day, so we were also sharing about our struggles. After awhile of doing this practice, we adjusted it to add two more terms. When something very awful happened, we called it a "sludge" event. When something extraordinarily wonderful happened, we designated it a "rainbow."

Susanne: From the very beginning, we made the commitment to find moments that made us laugh. Some days it was hard to do! But, we found humor in the devices they stuck on my husband's head, comments of nurses, and our own weird experiences. One particularly memorable time occurred after the tumor was first surgically removed, and my husband hadn't eaten solid food for 48 hours. He called me at home from the hospital early one morning to report he was reading a novel with a couple scene in it and delighted to notice feeling frisky in response. He called me back a few minutes later to say that a resident told him that the early biopsy report on the tumor showed it was likely cancerous. As I began asking him questions, he hung up on me, because his long-awaited breakfast of oatmeal showed up. I was angrier than I'd ever been at him, and upset about the cancer. I headed down to the hospital. Thankfully, a doctor was there who answered my questions and helped me calm down before walking into the hospital room. When I then had a conversation with my husband and let him know how angry I'd been, we began to see the humor in the situation. This became known in our relationship as our "horny, cancer, oatmeal moment"!

I often felt both a mix of happy and scared. My husband would come home from a hospital stay, which made me feel happy, but there was always some new medical procedure for me to learn to do. The family teased me about having dropped out of nursing school decades before, and to now be doing IV's and wound care. We would watch a movie, and I'd be distracted by watching to make sure my husband laughed enough, because it was good for him. I was happy to learn to manage our home and business finances, but very annoyed about the effort it took to do. We celebrated two wedding anniversaries in hospitals, which was grounds for both tears as well as joy that he was alive and we were together.

Practice in Action

Do one thing each day that makes you laugh, even if it's simply watching an old comedy re-run on TV.

Beneficial Character Strengths

Contentment is maintaining happiness and tranquility in body, mind, heart, and soul, with calm, accepting feelings and actions towards relationships, employment, surroundings, situations, and life in general.

Thankfulness is expressing warm, genuine feelings of praise, appreciation, and gratitude for such aspects of life as loved ones, blessings, benefits, lessons learned, challenges that prompt growth, and warm gestures.

10 - Spirit-Guided Choice:
DIE (AND LIVE) CONSCIOUSLY

The Concept

Many cancer patients regard thinking about dying as "giving up" or "being negative." They won't consider preparing for it or talking about it with their doctors or loved ones. Medical personnel and family may also resist or shut out the discussion. However, empowered healing requires consciously and courageously recognizing that while your prognosis is unknown, dying is a reality for everyone. It is simply the next stage in the life of your soul. This recognition may trigger appropriate grief for what you are facing in the time ahead and what you would be leaving behind and what you and your loved one would miss doing together. You may also be able to feel some happiness as you move through this final stage of your physical life and look forward, because death includes being free of disease and pain, and being in a better, spiritual place.

Preparing for the possibility of your passing away can also create healing acceptance of the totality of your life and celebration of your accomplishments. This life-review process has you and your loved ones examine the high points of your life and what you have done well. When you acknowledge to people that you know dying is possible in your circumstances, you may have to help them overcome denial. Facing reality provides opportunities for people to express to you directly what you have meant to them in the past and what you mean to them now.

As you think about your life and your funeral service, consider what fully honors the best of who you are and the work and service you have done. What family and friends do you want involved in your dying process and your funeral, and in what ways? What legacy do you want to leave behind? It may be helpful to think about any communications that you wish to create and give to someone for safekeeping. These could include such items as a letter for a child or grandchild for their graduation, birthday, religious event, or wedding day.

Engaging in the assessment of your life can also help you recognize what you have not done so you can take steps to accomplish the needed tasks. Remember, you can also ask someone else to help you do them. The goal is to feel "done" or "complete" with your life here. Achieving the maximum amount of healing of your mind, heart, and soul is vital, even when your body cannot heal in the way that you wanted or hoped.

When you courageously accept that dying is possible or likely, it creates a higher level of awareness of living each day as fully as you can and in the ways that you choose. The pace of each day can be more noble, quiet, and less frantic with activity. Or, you can do more activities than usual. You need not let go of your goal to live as long as possible. However, it is vital to consciously focus on the quality of your life. Each moment and each day is filled with choices. What choices will you make today that empower you?

Personal Perspectives

Craig: I reluctantly cooperated in making sure our estate documents were in order prior to the first tumor removal surgery. I refused to participate in funeral arrangements. I had no plans to die! After the tumor was removed a second time, we realized our estate documents were done incorrectly, and we had to fix them at a very high stress time. Thankfully, two of our relatives helped. A few months later, I realized that my wife was making funeral arrangements secretly, and it made no sense for her to do it alone. We had done many other projects in our marriage as partners, and this was one we could do together.

I ended up feeling very empowered by having significant input into what we ended up calling my end-of-life Honoring Service. The whole process of discovering what would honor me and my life resulted in compiling a book of my poetry, prose, and paintings over the years as well as creating a CD of my singing. We found videos that included me that we had never watched before, and we also watched the recording of our wedding. We had open discussions about what my wife's plans were after my passing. I was able to participate in discussions with friends about the soul and life after death, as well as what I was personally experiencing and feeling. I was able to reach a place of calmness and serenity about the possibility of dying. However, I still kept living one day at a time as best as I could.

Susanne: When I'm very anxious about something, I tend to focus on learning, planning, and orderliness. Faced with the prospect of my husband dying, I wanted to have everything in order, "just in case" something happened. I'm thankful that we had enough opportunities to get our legal paperwork and finances in order. I'm also very grateful that I got my husband's significant input into the funeral planning process before he lost the ability to communicate clearly. It also helped to have a good friend step in and agree to coordinate many of the planning details. A measure of grief accompanied each task, because it triggered the image of life without my husband. So, I turned to friends and my support group often to help express my thoughts and feelings.

A few weeks after my husband began hospice services, we decided to hold a large party in celebration of him and his life. We wanted people to have the opportunity to share directly with him how special he had been to them. Even with only two weeks advance notice, the party still drew over 200 people. It was a joyous occasion.

It was such a blessing to us and to so many others that we found recordings of my husband's voice and were able to put a music CD together. Finding his paintings from an art class taken a decade before was astounding. It was then a privilege that he let me read his journals and poetry and compile them into an amazing book. We had paintings and poetry framed together for our home that could also be displayed at the funeral/honoring service. The process of funeral planning was difficult at times, but it resulted in intimate moments for us and countless blessings. My husband's clear vision that he had a soul and that his soul would continue to live on gave him the confidence to approach death with a great deal of serenity, empowerment, and dignity.

We found that love, prayer, and the example of the hospice workers helped us to interact with my husband helpfully and respectfully, even when he could no longer talk or he seemed unconscious. We learned to observe and respond to his body signals and movements and to ask his permission or inform him before we did anything to or for him. We were able to then put cream on sore skin areas, start and stop pain medication, wash his itchy head, and hold his hand all in response to his physical signals and needs.

Practice in Action

When you have difficult tasks to do, such as visiting a funeral home to make arrangements, ensure that you have people you love go along with you.

Beneficial Character Strengths

Courage is taking brave and bold action, defending what is right, or facing and completing a worthwhile challenge, even when experiencing fear, resistance, uncertainty, opposition, hardship, or possible danger.

Wisdom is making good choices based upon knowledge gained from observation, education, and experiences, and reflecting and determining whether it is best to speak, remain silent, act, or be inactive.

RE-VISITING EMPOWERMENT

Our observation of society tells us that the world is shifting from an authoritarian model to one where people take responsibility for themselves. People are more willing and able to engage in consultative decision making rather than simply following orders. Doctors are no longer dictators of what is best for you and are your collaboration partners instead. When you integrate the fact-based and spirit-guided choices into your life and blend them together, they are aids in helping you engage in this collaboration process.

Remember that your ability to be an effective leader in responding to your cancer diagnosis requires you to make a commitment to maximize your quality of life. These insightful comments on commitment might help you with moving forward:

> The moment you believe you can do something, power seems to stream into you; the moment you believe you cannot do it, you have lost more than half the battle, you seem to be drained of the force necessary to do it.
> ~ Rúhíyyih Rabbani, *Prescription for Living* (1950 ed.), p. 39

> Until one is committed there is hesitancy, the chance to draw back, always ineffectiveness. Concerning all acts of initiative (and creation), there is one elementary truth, the ignorance of which kills countless ideas and splendid plans: that the moment one definitely commits oneself, then Providence moves too. All sorts of things occur to help one that would never

otherwise have occurred. A whole stream of events issues from the decision, raising in one's favor all manner of unforeseen incidents and meetings and material assistance, which no man could have dreamt would have come his way.
>   ~ W. H. Murray, *The Scottish Himalayan Expedition*, pp. 6-7

Facing cancer and dealing with everything associated with it is not easy. These experiences will likely include some of the more difficult moments of your life. Our request is to move past the paralysis that fear brings and step into effective action. Consider this:

> Even though possibilities always exist, we lose sight of them when we are blinded by fear. ... When this happens, our problem-solving creativity shrivels. At worst, it narrows to just fighting, fleeing, and freezing. We become merely reactive instead of proactive. Problems become prisons.
>
> Freedom from these self-imposed prisons comes only when we suspend fear by evoking appreciation, envisioning all of our remaining possibilities, and then choosing one.
>
> Choice is proactivity, and choice is power. It charts the course of our lives. It makes us happy.
>   ~ Dan Baker, PhD, and Cameron Stauth, *What Happy People Know: How the New Science of Happiness Can Change Your Life for the Better*, pp. 116-117

We wish you well on your fact-based, spirit-guided cancer journey and with the choices that you make!

~ Susanne and Craig

Appendix A: COPY OF "THREE TOOLS OF HEALING" POSTER

Designed and copyrighted by Justice St Rain,
www.interfaithresources.com.

THREE TOOLS OF HEALING

From the Sacred Writings of the Bahá'í Faith

MEDICAL TREATMENT

"There are two ways of healing sickness, material means and spiritual means. The first is by the treatment of physicians,...

PRAYER

"the second consisteth in prayers offered by the spiritual ones to God and in turning to Him. Both means should be used and practiced."

"The prayers which were revealed to ask for healing apply both to physical and spiritual healing. Recite them, then, to heal both the soul and the body."

JOY & LAUGHTER

"...thou shouldst impart gladness to thy patient, give him comfort and joy, and bring him to ecstasy and exultation. How often hath it occurred that this hath caused early recovery."

"When at the bedside of a patient, cheer and gladden his heart and enrapture his spirit through celestial power. Indeed, such a heavenly breath quickeneth every mouldering bone and reviveth the spirit of every sick and ailing one."

Thy name is my healing, O my God, and remembrance of Thee is my remedy.
Nearness to Thee is my hope, and love for Thee is my companion.
Thy mercy to me is my healing and my succor in both this world and the world to come.
Thou, verily, art the All-Bountiful, the All-Knowing, the All-Wise.
- A Bahá'í Prayer for Healing -

©1998 Justice St Rain

Appendix B: EMPOWERING CHARACTER QUALITIES

Simply put, **character is:**
- The sum of all the qualities you develop throughout your life as you make choices about how to speak and act; character affects the majority of your words and actions
- The spiritual essence of who you are as a human being
- Your moral compass or ethical strength that provides the unwavering drive to choose what is right, even when that choice could cause you difficulties, and even if no one else is watching you or knows what you are doing

The character qualities below are some that most influence interpersonal relationships and marriages. You may find it helpful to choose certain ones to strengthen as you make fact-based, spirit-guided cancer choices and choose empowered healing.

1. **Acceptance is** a deep, meaningful embracing of who someone is, as well as acknowledging that people and events are as they are, or were as they were, rather than wasting time and energy trying to change people, regret the past, or influence events when it is unwise or there is no possibility of success.
2. **Assertiveness is** speaking up or acting decisively to improve a situation for the benefit of others and oneself.
3. **Beauty is** expressing the best of one's inner spirit and demonstrating, seeing, and creating attractiveness, loveliness, or order wherever possible.
4. **Caring is** giving sincere love, attention, consideration, and assistance to others and responding to needy situations in timely and appropriate ways.

5. **Chastity is** maintaining sexual purity and reserving sexual attraction, responses, and intimacy as a special and respectful gift to share with a marriage partner.
6. **Commitment is** making and keeping a reasonable promise or binding agreement to others or to oneself, including setting and meeting certain goals, standards, or expectations, as well as completing tasks to which one has agreed.
7. **Compassion is** feeling genuine concern for others and oneself, empathizing with the pain and suffering of those in difficult situations, and seeking ways to relieve their pain and ease their suffering.
8. **Confidence is** trusting one's inner value, worthy intentions, capacity to think and act effectively, and ability to accomplish stated goals of oneself and of others.
9. **Contentment is** maintaining happiness and tranquility in body, mind, heart, and soul, with calm, accepting feelings and actions towards relationships, employment, surroundings, situations, and life in general.
10. **Cooperation is** working with others in harmony to create or accomplish something that would be more difficult or impossible to accomplish by one person working alone.
11. **Courage is** taking brave and bold action, defending what is right, or facing and completing a worthwhile challenge, even when experiencing fear, resistance, uncertainty, opposition, hardship, or possible danger.
12. **Courtesy is** showing gracious and warm consideration for others by interacting with polite manners, respectful gestures, thoughtful actions, and kind language.
13. **Creativity is** drawing on ideas, inspiration, or imagination to develop or produce something new, including contributions and solutions that benefit others.
14. **Detachment is** stepping back to gain a different perspective on what is happening and placing less importance on

worldly concerns, while selflessly letting go of one's feelings, hopes, desires, attachments, and need to be in control.
15. **Discernment is** perceiving and understanding oneself, others, and situations accurately and objectively, including discriminating between what is beneficial and what is harmful, without prejudice or bias.
16. **Encouragement is** offering sincere, uplifting acknowledgment of the character strengths, effective actions, or good intentions of others and oneself; inspiring or assisting others and oneself to start, continue, or stop doing something; and fostering personal growth and development.
17. **Enthusiasm is** expressing genuine positive and joyful feelings, often in a high-spirited way, about an occasion, activity, important occurrence, goal, person, or extraordinary situation.
18. **Equality is** creating a balanced partnership between people who work together as a team, especially a woman and man in a relationship or marriage, respecting each person as a worthy and noble human being.
19. **Excellence is** striving to achieve high standards and a superior quality of work and effort, as well as fulfilling one's potential for character growth and development.
20. **Faithfulness is** being steadfast and maintaining commitments to others, to a set of beliefs, or to an organization.
21. **Flexibility is** adjusting to life as it happens and embracing changes as needed, while remaining true to one's core values, beliefs, and appropriate priorities.
22. **Forgiveness is** pardoning someone for saying or doing something hurtful or harmful, giving up a desire for revenge, and letting go of anger and resentment.
23. **Fortitude is** staying brave, resolute, steadfast, and strong mentally, emotionally, physically, and spiritually when

— Appendix B: Empowering Character Qualities —

facing challenges, difficulties, adversity, danger, pain, or temptation.
24. **Friendliness is** demonstrating an outgoing and positive social attitude and reaching out to connect with and build relationships with people.
25. **Generosity is** giving away or sharing what one has, such as affection, money, time, appreciation, encouragement, gifts, celebrations, positive feedback, resources, knowledge, wisdom, possessions, physical abilities, personal energy, ideas, or resources with open mind, heart, and hands.
26. **Gentleness is** expressing consideration from the heart, honoring the feelings of others and oneself, and using soft and careful physical touch, movement, and words.
27. **Helpfulness is** taking appropriate action to address the needs or participate in solving the problems of others or oneself.
28. **Honesty is** acting and speaking consistently with high and incorruptible moral, ethical, and legal standards.
29. **Humility is** seeing the strengths, imperfections, abilities, accomplishments, failures, and all other aspects of oneself and others in realistic perspective; acting consistently according to principles, morals, and values rather than ego; and acknowledging the greatness of God.
30. **Idealism is** envisioning what is possible, thinking beyond what currently exists, and taking action towards or advocating for beneficial change.
31. **Integrity is** achieving a state of balance and wholeness in life and character, by acting in accord with civil laws and deepest beliefs, highest values and principles, and stated word.
32. **Joyfulness is** being in a state of high-spirited and ecstatic delight, gladness, blissfulness, great happiness, and jubilation.

33. **Justice is** making a fair decision or taking fair action free of any bias or prejudice after carefully assessing all the facts, feelings, people, principles, laws, risks, and consequences related to a situation.
34. **Kindness is** considering the needs or wants of others and acting in a deliberately warm-hearted and empathetic manner to meet them.
35. **Love is** connecting to others through affection and joining with them to express the powerfully magnetic and caring force that unites the universe.
36. **Loyalty is** honoring, belonging to, supporting, and remaining devoted and faithful to someone or something beyond oneself; such as, a friend, partner, spouse, family, employers, organizations, community, religion, country, or the world.
37. **Mercy is** treating the mistakes or harmful actions of others in a forbearing and lenient way.
38. **Moderation is** recognizing and avoiding extremes in use of time, words, actions, and other choices, to seek a balance that creates positive outcomes.
39. **Patience is** maintaining steady awareness and control of one's thoughts and responses while waiting for or seeking an outcome; controlling one's words and actions while willingly and calmly taking the time to respond to difficult, inconvenient, hurtful, delaying, or troublesome situations.
40. **Peacefulness is** being physically, mentally, and emotionally calm and serene and working to reduce conflict and build harmony between people.
41. **Perseverance is** persisting and pressing onward towards worthwhile goals, particularly in the face of challenges or adversity.
42. **Purity is** maintaining personal physical cleanliness, a clean and orderly environment, uplifting and chaste

— Appendix B: Empowering Character Qualities —

thoughts, positive words, honest motivations, a loving heart, and a spiritually focused soul.
43. **Purposefulness is** pursuing meaningful goals and participating in vital activities with determination.
44. **Resilience is** accepting, responding appropriately to, recovering from, and coping with adversity, misfortune, change, or illness, and bouncing back from stressful experiences effectively and in a reasonable amount of time.
45. **Respect is** interacting with all people and what they value, as well as animals and the environment, in a manner that demonstrates they are worthy of fair treatment, consideration, and honorable regard.
46. **Responsibility is** claiming personal accountability for one's own life, choices, happiness, commitments, required activities, and relationships with others, as well as sharing accountability for the quality of life in the communities in which one lives and works and the global society.
47. **Self-Discipline is** maintaining the inner control to perform needed and important tasks; fulfill one's commitments, goals, and life purposes; and resist what is harmful to others or oneself.
48. **Service is** acting selflessly and often sacrificially, directly or indirectly, to improve or enhance the well-being and quality of life of others and their situations and experiences.
49. **Sincerity is** being genuine and earnest about one's motives, words, and actions.
50. **Spirituality is** nurturing your heart and soul through maintaining a close, interactive relationship with God, drawing on spiritual sources for divine guidance, dedicated or devoted to the service of God or religion, and acting and speaking in alignment with the teachings in the Word of God.

51. **Tactfulness is** choosing whether and when to act or speak and, when speaking, using gentle and kind words with the intention of not offending others or hurting their feelings.
52. **Thankfulness is** expressing warm, genuine feelings of praise, appreciation, and gratitude for such aspects of life as loved ones, blessings, benefits, lessons learned, challenges that prompt growth, and warm gestures.
53. **Thoughtfulness is** being concerned in a deliberate and genuine way about the well-being and happiness of others, acting in anticipation of and in loving awareness of their needs.
54. **Thriftiness is** managing ones economic situation and expenditures in a wise and frugal way to meet needs adequately, create prosperity, and successfully plan positive outcomes.
55. **Trustworthiness is** handling tasks, responsibilities, possessions, money, and information reliably and honestly, thereby earning the confidence of others.
56. **Truthfulness is** communicating accurately to convey one's best understanding of facts and feelings.
57. **Unity is** consciously looking for and strengthening points of commonality, harmony, and attraction, as well as working with others to build a strong foundation of oneness, love, commitment, and cooperation.
58. **Wisdom is** making good choices based upon knowledge gained from observation, education, and experiences, and reflecting and determining whether it is best to speak, remain silent, act, or be inactive.

ABOUT THE AUTHORS

Susanne M. Alexander and *Craig A. Farnsworth* married in August 1999, a second marriage for both of them. Between them, they have four adult children and three grandchildren. Both Susanne and Craig are members of the Bahá'í Faith (**www.bahai.org**).

Susanne and Craig trained as relationship and marriage coaches and educators with a specialty in character. They facilitated marriage preparation and marriage enrichment workshops with people of all ages together. Susanne and Craig founded Marriage Transformation LLC, which empowers people globally to create happy, lasting, character-based marriages (**www.marriagetransformation.com; www.bahaimarriage.net**). Their first book, published in 2003, was *Marriage Can Be Forever—Preparation Counts!* They subsequently created *Pure Gold: Encouraging Character Qualities in Marriage.* Susanne has since authored or coauthored many books to empower people to have excellent relationships and marriages.

Susanne is a workshop leader, public speaker, and freelance journalist. She has a BA in Communications from Baldwin-Wallace College in Ohio. She is a member of the American Society of Journalists and Authors and Toastmasters International. Her over 200 articles have been published in **www.yourtango.com, www.simplemarriage.net, www.parentsconnect.com**, *Newsweek Japan, The (Cleveland) Plain Dealer, Crain's Cleveland Business,* and *Massage Magazine* among others. She has been quoted as an expert in many publications and on the radio. Details are available at **www.marriagetransformation.com/speaking.htm** and **www.marriagetransformation.com/aboutus_mediacoverage.htm**.

Prior to his passing of brain cancer on July 1, 2009, *Craig* was a market manager for Radix Wire Company. He earned BA degrees in Physics and Elementary Education from Hiram College in Ohio. He taught elementary school for four years before becoming a gas appliance research and developer. He had technical articles published in a variety of industry publications. He was a member of the American Society of Gas Engineers and served on the steering committee for the International Appliance Technical Conference.

Craig was a musician, playing many types of flutes and the guitar. He sang bass in choirs, and he performed in the United States and Canada with the Voices of Bahá choir, including performing in Carnegie Hall.

Craig's commitment was to make a difference for others, truly living to serve. He was a VIP Hero blood donor for the American Red Cross, on the school board for his local Bahá'í Sunday school, on various Bahá'í committees including for an annual youth conference, facilitated Honest Conversations race dialogue sessions, coached others through building community change projects, was active in Toastmasters, and served on the boards of directors and as an officer for the Interfaith Suburban Action Coalition, Euclid Community Concerns, Better Together marriage coalition, and his neighborhood association.

PLEASE CONTACT US

We welcome hearing from you about your experiences with this book and having you **purchase additional copies** for friends and relatives. Please share anything about how *Empowered Healing* has helped you, as well as any **feedback** that would improve its usefulness for others. Remember Marriage Transformation is also willing to work with you on using the book for **fundraising** initiatives.

Contact Information

Marriage Transformation LLC
Susanne M. Alexander,
President; Relationship & Marriage Coach;
Character Development Specialist
Cleveland, Ohio, USA

E-mail:

Susanne@marriagetransformation.com
or staff@marriagetransformation.com
Skype: MarriageTransformation

Websites:

www.marriagetransformation.com
www.bahaimarriage.net; www.bahairelationships.com
www.allinonemarriageprep.com
www.marriagetransformation.com/store_EmpowercdHealing.htm

Social Media:

www.twitter.com/Marriage4ever
www.facebook.com/MarriageTransformation
www.linkedin.com/in/susannemalexander

Please be sure to visit our website **to purchase an ever-growing selection of exciting new books, eBooks, coaching services, and training materials.** Sets of worksheets from various books are also often available for purchase through: **www.marriagetransformation.com/store.htm.**

Please **subscribe**, on our websites, to our free e-newsletter, which has great articles and information for you about relationships, marriage, new books, and book sales. Our books are also often available through your favorite distributor or a local or on-line bookseller!

Speaking:

Susanne M. Alexander, professional speaker and author, can also be scheduled to speak at events or to present workshops for individuals, couples, professionals, patients, and caregivers.

Susanne's dynamic speaking presentations and interactive workshops include stories of real experiences and strategies shared with compassion, inspiration, and humor. Please contact Susanne today to discuss your needs and to schedule a presentation or workshop.

www.marriagetransformation.com/speaking.htm

www.ingramcontent.com/pod-product-compliance
Lightning Source LLC
Chambersburg PA
CBHW051454290426
44109CB00016B/1756